Practical Retinal Photography and Digital Imaging Techniques

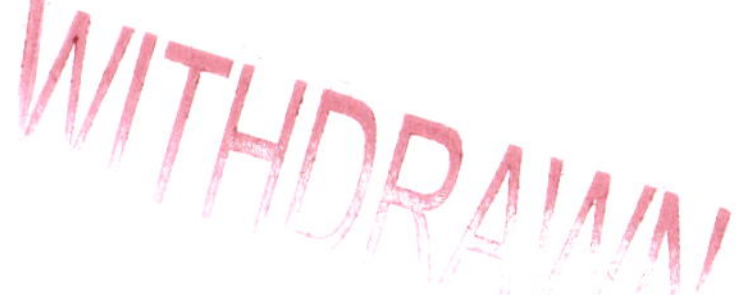

Practical Retinal Photography and Digital Imaging Techniques

Marshall E. Tyler, CRA, FOPS
Instructor, Surgical Sciences (Ophthalmology)
Department of Ophthalmology
Wake Forest University Medical Center
Winston-Salem, North Carolina

Patrick J. Saine, MEd, CRA, FOPS
Instructor of Surgery (Ophthalmology)
Dartmouth Medical School
Manager, Ophthalmic Photography
Section of Ophthalmology
Dartmouth-Hitchcock Medical Center
Lebanon, New Hampshire

Timothy J. Bennett, CRA, FOPS
Senior Ophthalmic Photographer
Ophthalmology Department
Penn State Milton S. Hershey Medical Center
Hershey, Pennsylvania

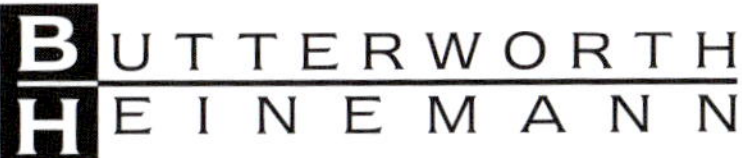

An Imprint of Elsevier Science

BUTTERWORTH-HEINEMANN
An Imprint of Elsevier Science (USA)

The Curtis Center
Independence Square West
Philadelphia, Pennsylvania 19106

NOTICE

Ophthalmology is an ever-changing field. Standard safety precautions must be followed but as new research and clinical experience broaden our knowledge, changes in treatment and drug therapy may become necessary or appropriate. Readers are advised to check the most current product information provided by the manufacturer of each drug to be administered to verify the recommended dose, the method and duration of administration, and contraindications. It is the responsibility of the treating physician, relying on experience and knowledge of the patient, to determine dosages and the best treatment for each individual patient. Neither the Publisher nor the author assumes any liability for any injury and/or damage to persons or property arising from this publication.

The Publisher

The photo-illustration on the cover was created by Patrick Saine from an original black and white digital fundus photograph, using Photoshop on a Macintosh computer.

Library of Congress Cataloging in Publication Data

Tyler, Marshall E.
    Practical retinal photography and digital imaging techniques/Marshall E. Tyler, Patrick J. Saine, Timothy J. Bennett.—1st ed.
       p. cm.
    Includes bibliographical references and index.
    ISBN 0-7506-7371-0
    1. Retina–Imaging. 2. Ophthalmic photography. I. Saine, Patrick J. II. Bennett, T. J. (Timothy J.) III. Title.
    RE551 .T95 2003
    617.7′350754—dc21
                                          2002038413

Editor: Natasha Andjelkovic
Editorial Assistant: Danielle Burke

RDC/WAL

Printed in the United States of America

Last digit is the print number: 9 8 7 6 5 4 3 2 1

Contents

Contents

We are witnessing the expansion of retinal photography beyond the traditional clinical and research use of 35 mm slides. Nontraditional settings represent one recent trend. Nonmydriatic cameras are found in increasing numbers in optometrists' offices. Endrocinologist-based screening of diabetic retinopathy is gaining favor, and a large number of newer drug studies utilize fundus photography to monitor patient changes. The production of fundus images in these settings indicates that ophthalmic photography is no longer being practiced solely by photographically trained individuals in specialists' offices.

The purpose of this book is to provide a resource for professionals whose roles require quality retinal imaging but whose education does not include photographic training. Fundus photography is an introduction to the larger field of ophthalmic photography. This book contains step-by-step procedures for the novice fundus photographer and shares the techniques required to produce sharp, well-focused retinal photographs.

A second trend is imaging's steady march from silver-based to silicon-based media. Newer fundus cameras, both traditional and nonmydriatic, now provide digital images as output. Older film-based fundus cameras are being converted to digital imaging systems, and both film and flatbed scanners are being used to import extant patient slides and prints into the digital medium. But this is only half of the equation. Once the ophthalmic image is in the computer, how can we share it—"re-purpose it" to use the lingo—either via e-mail or within a computer-based presentation? How do we transfer the images to a web page PowerPoint presentation, or a printed report? This book will familiarize you with successful strategies for taking full advantage of the digital medium.

We think of this book as a stepping stone. It is a step beyond point and shoot; a step toward understanding the complexity of a photographic medium that includes ocular angiography, anterior segment photography, and media production. We encourage you to move beyond the basic information presented here and to fully explore the ophthalmic photography experience.

Marshall E. Tyler, CRA, FOPS
Patrick J. Saine, MEd, CRA, FOPS
Timothy J. Bennett, CRA, FOPS

Acknowledgments

We would like to thank the physicians with whom we work for encouraging our professional growth by supporting our ophthalmic photography writing and publication projects. An invigorating clinical ophthalmic photography setting exists in each of our workplaces. We acknowledge M. Madison Slusher, MD, The Richard G. Weaver Professor of Surgery and Chairman of the Department of Ophthalmology at Wake Forest University School of Medicine; Rosalind A. Stevens, MD, Chief of Ophthalmology at Dartmouth Medical School; and David A. Quillen, MD, and George W. Blankenship, MD, the current and former Chairman of the Department of Ophthalmology at the Penn State Milton S. Hershey Medical Center.

We are grateful to all of the ophthalmic photographers who have shared their expertise with us, either personally or through the Internet discussion group Optimal. We thank the Ophthalmic Photographers' Society as an institution that provides a forum for the exploration of all that is new in ophthalmic imaging. Specifically, a thank you to Leslie MacKeen, Gary Michalec, and Richard Hackel for supplying images for figures.

We graciously thank Natasha Andjelkovic and Karen Oberheim of Butterworth-Heinemann for their encouragement and support on this project. We thank Peggy Gordon of P. M. Gordon Associates for her editorial expertise.

We thank our families for their understanding. Thank you Alix and Christina; Deb, Julie, and Beth; and Ellen and Emily for supporting our ambitions.

No matter how slow the film,
spirit always stands still long enough
for the photographer it has chosen.
—*Minor White*

The Basics
History, Basic Eye Anatomy, and the Fundus Camera

The word *photography* literally means "writing with light." Paradoxically, in performing fundus photography, the subject of light's picture essay is the very structure we use to perceive that light. This chapter provides a basic grounding in the material required to master fundus photography. We will start with some history, review basic eye anatomy, and then look closely at the instrument called the fundus camera. Read this chapter if you are new to eye care or have never examined a patient's retina.

A Short History of Fundus Photography

The first published account of in vivo human retinal photography is by Jackman and Webster in 1886[1] (Fig. 1–1). An albo-carbon light source provided illumination during the 2½-minute exposure. As important as these early attempts were, the images were quite blurry.

High-quality fundus photography began at the turn of the twentieth century with the work of Frederick Dimmer. Arthur Bedell wrote that Dimmer "electrified the 9th International Congress (1899) with his marvelous pictures...."[2] Dimmer's 1907 treatise on fundus photography described his cumbersome apparatus, which used carbon arc illumination (Fig. 1–2).[3] He was the first to incorporate fundus photography into a basic ophthalmic textbook and the first to publish a photographic atlas.[4,5]

Color fundus photography was described as early as 1929, the same year Bedell published the first stereo atlas of fundus photographs.[6] In 1946, Harold Edgerton developed the electronic flash tube,[7] and in 1949 Rizzutti introduced

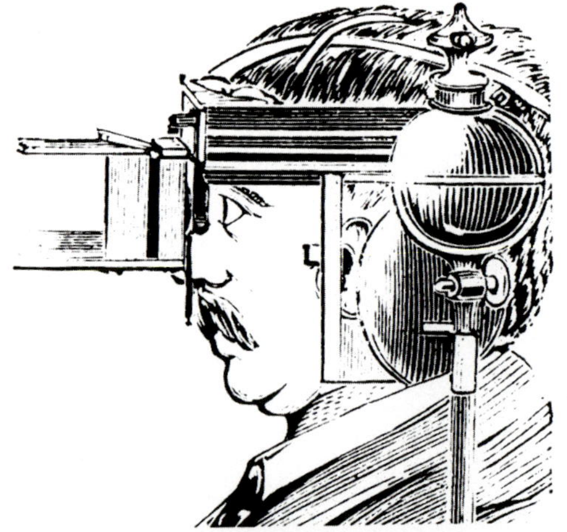

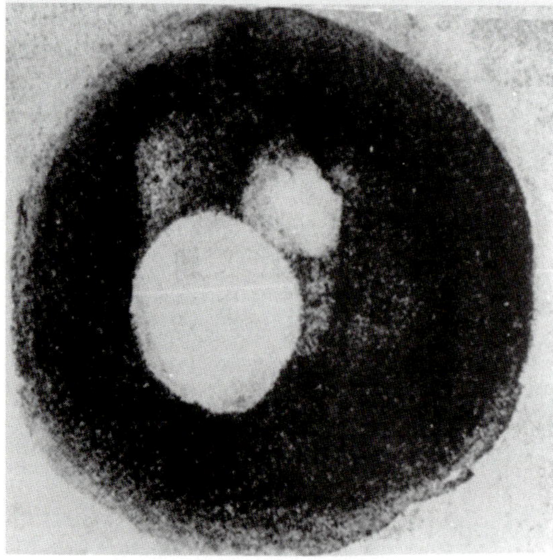

Figure 1–1 ○ *Top,* Jackman and Webster produced the first published human fundus photograph using an albo-carbon burner, an ophthalmoscopic mirror, and a 2$\frac{1}{2}$-minute exposure. *Bottom,* Interpretation requires some imagination: The small upper white area is the optic disc, and the lower, larger light area is an artifact. Blood vessels cannot be defined. (Reprinted with permission from WA Mann: History of photography of the eye. *Surv Ophthal* 1970;15:179.)

its use to ophthalmology.[8] Electronic flash was adapted to the fundus camera in 1953 in both Britain and the United States (Fig. 1–3)[9,10]

Wide-angle fundus cameras were introduced in the 1970s, nonmydriatic cameras in the 1980s, and mainstream scanning laser ophthalmoscopes in the 1990s. Like the rest of the imaging world today, fundus photography is participating in the digital revolution.

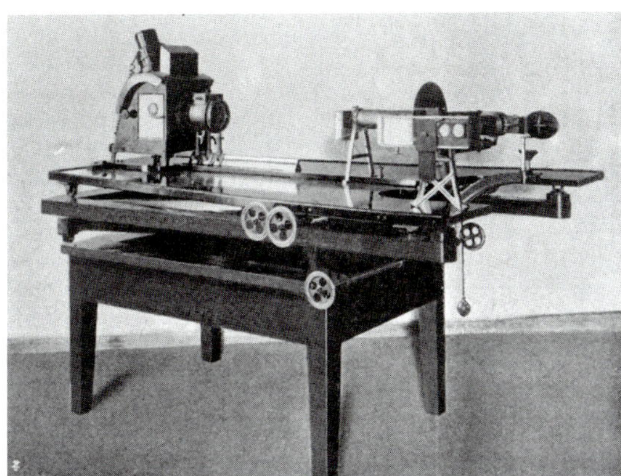

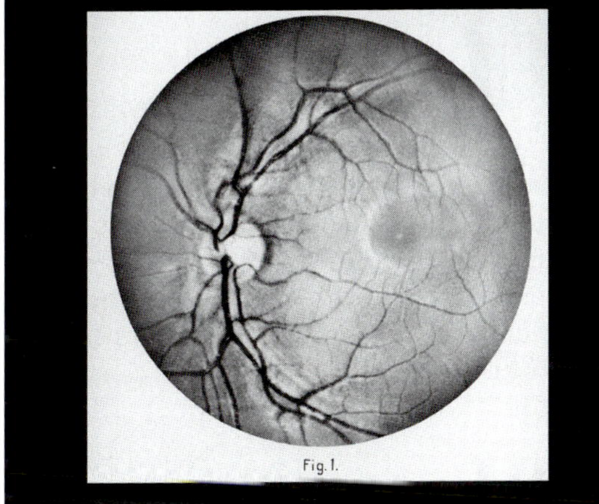

Figure 1–2 ○ Dimmer's fundus camera (*top*) was used to create the first fine retinal photographs such as this normal eye (*bottom*). (Reprinted from Pes O: La Photographie du fond de l'oeil. Turin: Vincenzo Bona, 1906; and F. Dimmer: Demonstration von Photogrammen Des Augernhintergrundes. Wiesbaden, Germany: Verlag von J.F. Bergmann, 1903.)

Basic Eye Anatomy

This basic overview will help you orient yourself during fundus photography (Fig. 1–4). It is not meant to take the place of a thorough study of an ocular anatomy text in which the eye's development, histology, and function are fully described.[11,12]

The eye is the sense organ of sight (Fig. 1–5). Measuring about 24 mm in diameter, it is protected by the bones of the orbit and moves with the help of six extraocular muscles. The rapidly blinking eyelid and tough sclera protect the eye's contents.

Light enters the eye through the cornea, then moves through the lens and vitreous (a clear, gelatinous mass composed of 98.8% water that helps the eye hold its shape) toward the retina. The cornea and lens combine to refract light

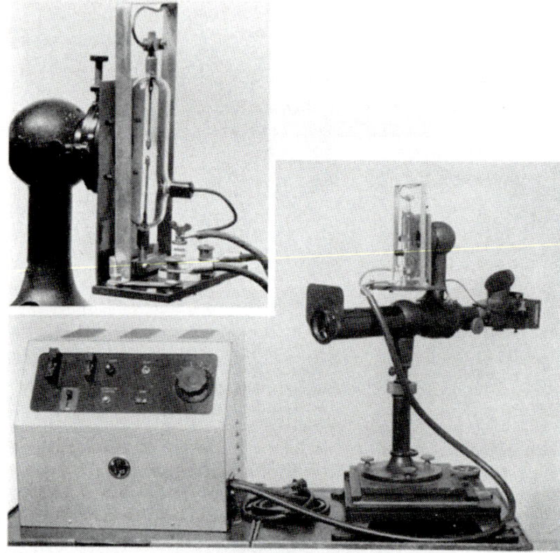

Figure 1–3 ○ Hansell and Beeson adapted the electronic flash tube to a Zeiss fundus camera. (Reprinted with permission from Hansell P: *A System of Ophthalmic Illustration.* Springfield: Charles C Thomas, 1957.)

whose focus is the retina. The lens is suspended by thin zonules. Stimulated by light that reaches the retina, the iris expands and contracts to enlarge or reduce the size of the pupil. This automatic exposure mechanism adjusts the amount of light that falls on the retina. Another important anterior chamber structure is the ciliary body, which produces the aqueous fluid that fills the anterior chamber. This fluid drains from the eye through the filtration angle and Schlemm's canal.

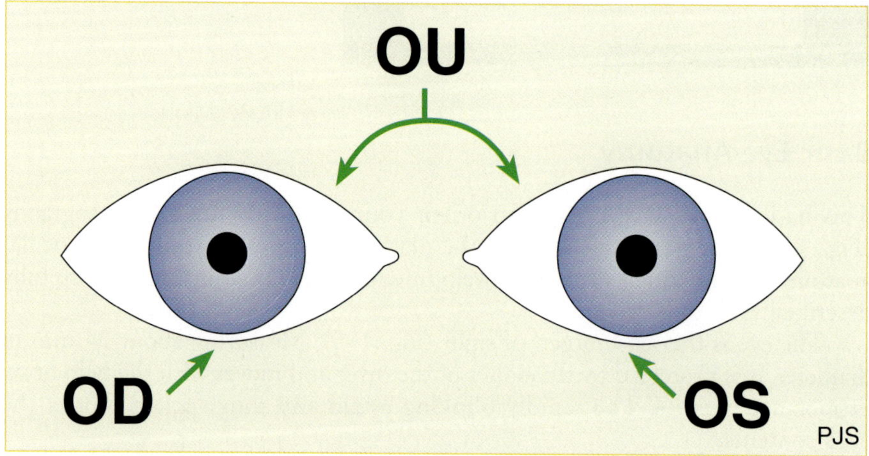

Figure 1–4 ○ When referring to both eyes together, the abbreviation OU (ocular uterque or ocular uniti) is used. The right eye is labeled OD (ocular dexter), and the left eye OS (ocular sinister).

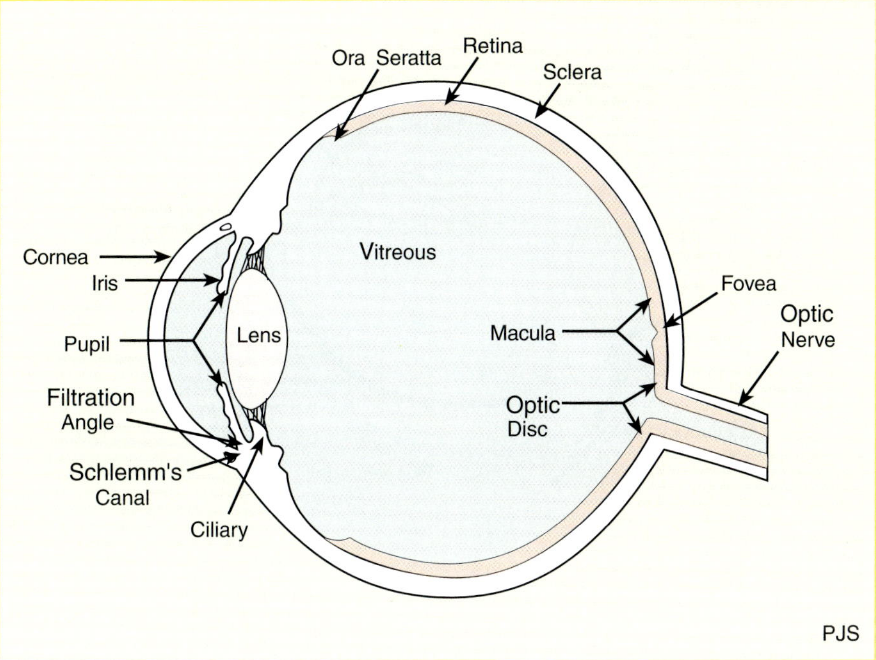

Figure 1–5 ○ A cross section of the eye, showing the major ocular structures with which each fundus photographer should be familiar.

The retina is a multilayered membrane measuring from 0.10 to 0.23 mm thick. It transforms light energy into chemical impulses that travel to the brain through the optic nerve. The retina is nourished by two sets of blood vessels: the retinal blood vessels and the choroidal blood vessels (Fig. 1–6). The central retinal artery, a branch of the ophthalmic artery, enters the globe through the optic nerve. It branches into the outbound retinal arteries (thinner, lighter blood vessels) and returning retinal veins (thicker, darker blood vessels). The choroid describes a network of spongy blood vessels that are separated from the retina by a layer of pigmented cells called the retinal pigment epithelium (RPE).

The retina is transparent. When we look at a normal fundus photograph, we see the red retinal arteries and retinal veins superimposed on an orange background that is the choroid as filtered by the coloration of the RPE.

Central reading vision occurs in the important retinal landmarks of the fovea and macula. Histologically, the fovea describes a small (0.5 mm) central depression that contains the richest saturation of cones. Through a fundus camera, you can more easily discern a centrally located area of darker xanthophyll pigmentation termed the macula.

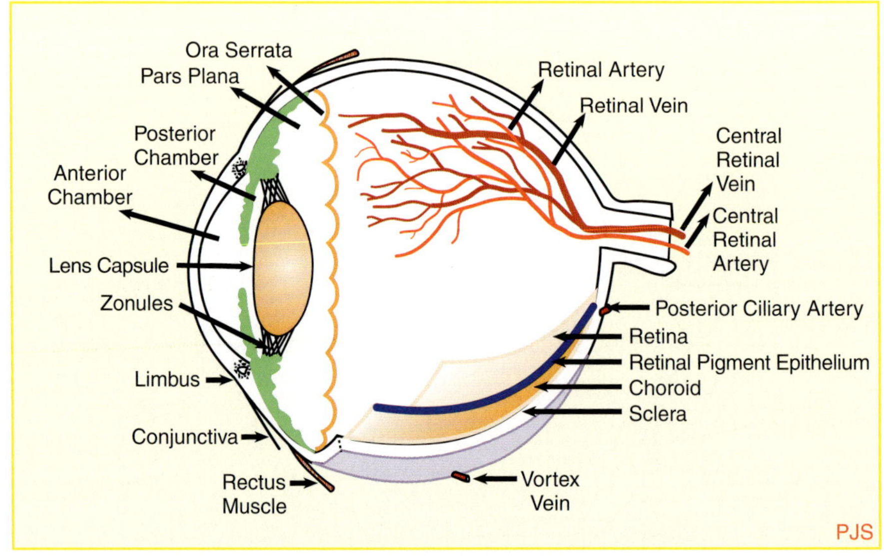

Figure 1–6 ○ Note the layered aspect of the retina.

The curving course of these blood vessels forms the inferior and superior arcades (Fig. 1–7). The central area contained within these arcades is termed the posterior pole. On the outside of these blood vessels is the periphery: the closer midperiphery and the far periphery near the ora serrata. The outer edge of the retina, the ora serrata, is beyond the reach of most fundus cameras. Anterior means front, while posterior refers to the back of the eye. Superior and inferior label up and down. Nasal refers to the nose, while temporal refers to the temples.

Measurements within the fundus are often approximated in disc diameters (DD) (Fig. 1–8). For example, the fovea usually lies about 2.5 DD temporal and slightly inferior to the midline of the optic disc. Clock hours and the seven standard retinal fields are also used to describe locations within the retinal landscape.

Are you unsure as to which area of the retina you are viewing or have photographed? When in doubt, visualize the position of the optic nerve. As with all roads and Rome, all retinal blood vessel bifurcations lead back to the optic nerve (Fig. 1–9).

The Fundus Camera

The camera is like an eye. It is basically a light-tight box (globe = camera body) that focuses light (lens + cornea = camera lens) onto a receiving plane (retina = film). A cover (eyelid = shutter) determines when light enters the box.

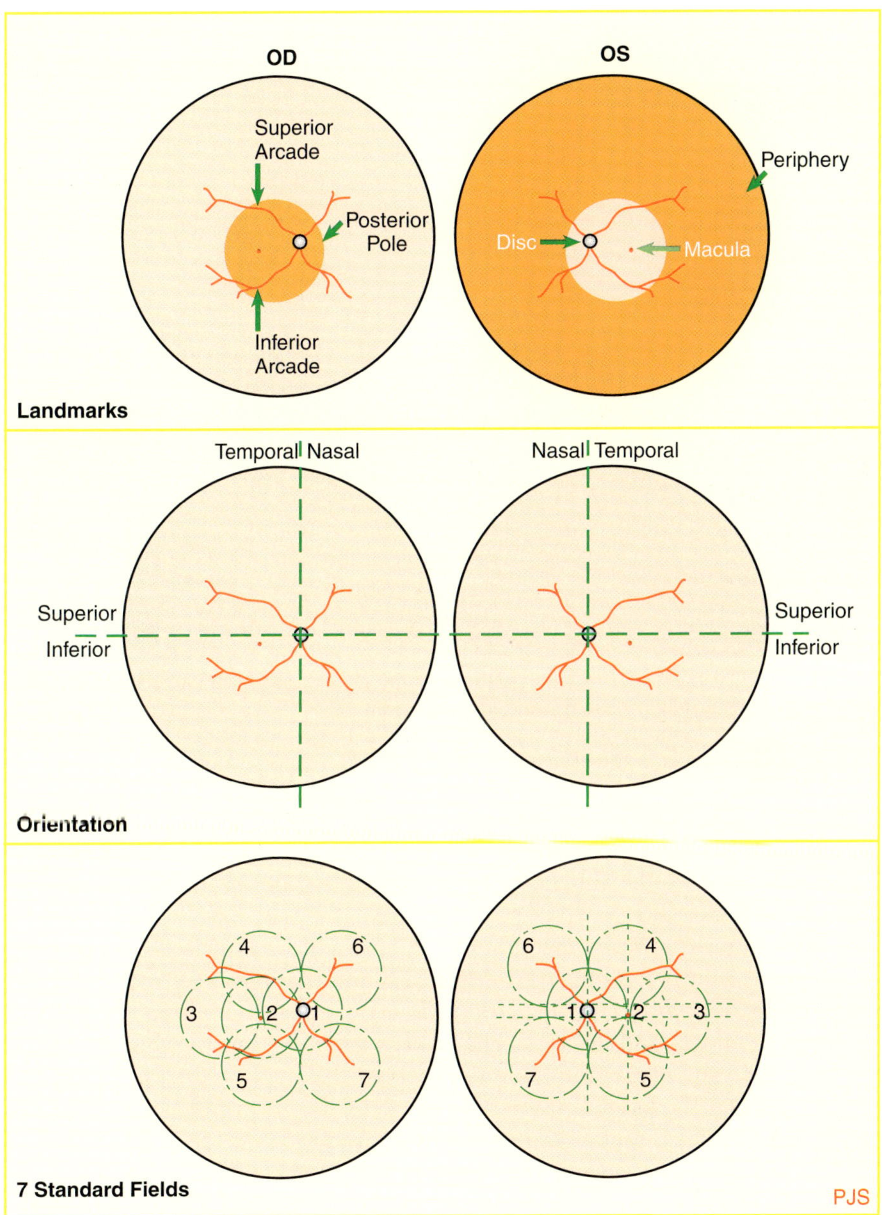

Figure 1–7 ◯ Landmarks: A retinal lesion may be located in the posterior pole (the disc, macula, and the area enclosed within the inferior and superior arcades) or within the periphery (the area outside of the arcades). Orientation: Directions, such as temporal (toward the temple), nasal (toward the nose), inferior, and superior, allow greater specificity. Seven Standard Fields: The seven standard fields describe specific retinal locations as imaged by a 30-degree fundus camera. Clock hours can also be used to specify location.

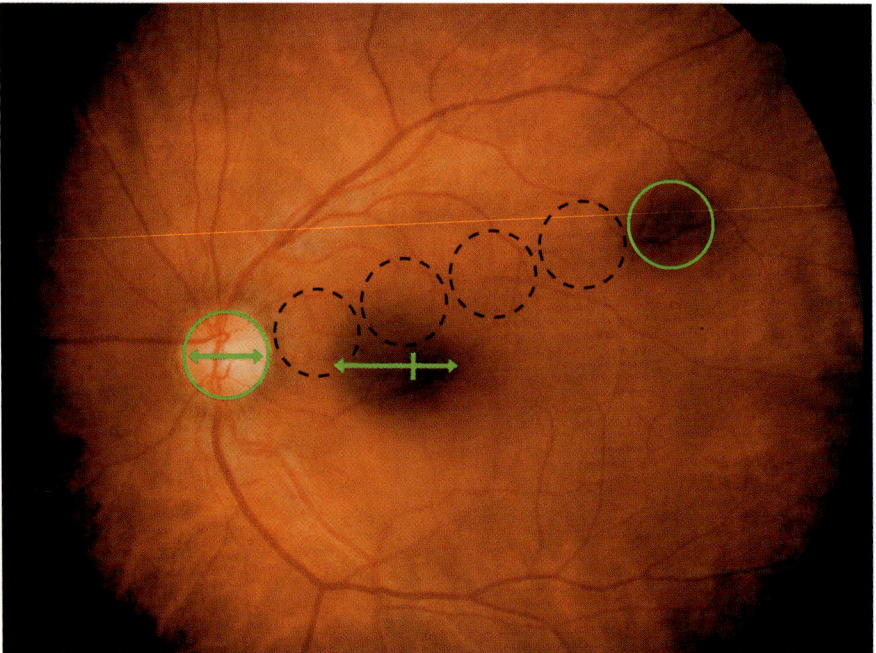

Figure 1–8 ○ Disc diameter (the width of the optic nerve) is a convenient intraocular measuring stick. In a normal patient, the macula lies approximately 2.5 disc diameters temporal to the disc and just below a line that bisects the disc. The nevus located 5 disc diameters superior and temporal to the optic nerve measures about 1 disc diameter.

The optical instrument that is used to document the visual condition of the retina is called a fundus camera. It is a specialized low-power microscope with an attached camera.

All automobiles have a steering wheel, an engine, and wheels. The steering wheel guides you, the engine provides energy, and the wheels get you where you want to go. Likewise, all *fundus cameras* share three interrelated subsystems: mechanical, optical, and electrical. The joystick steers the camera, while the optical system creates the image from light energy provided by the electrical system.

Support for the fundus camera is provided by the mechanical subsystem. The heavy optical head is mounted on a height-adjustable table, the most versatile of which is wheelchair accessible. The chinrest and forehead rest minimize patient head movement. During the procedure, precise positioning is controlled by the joystick and optical head height control.

The retinal image is transferred to the film by using the optical subsystem. The classic fundus camera design features an aspheric objective lens precisely aligned with a 35-mm single-lens reflex camera body (Fig. 1–10). Simply stated,

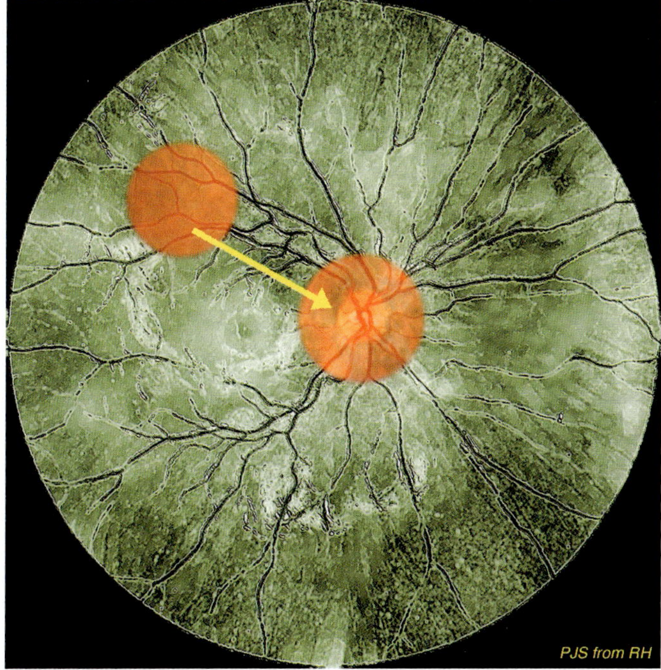

Figure 1–9 ○ If you are unsure where in the retina a field is located, consider a vessel bifurcation to be an arrow that points toward the optic nerve.

the optical system of the fundus camera projects a ring of illumination through the dilated pupil; the light then reflects off the retina, exits the pupil through the center of the illumination ring, and continues through the fundus camera optics to form an image at the film plane. The viewfinder and the film back or digital recording device are integral parts of this subsystem.

The electrical subsystem powers two illumination sources (Fig. 1–11). Viewing the retina requires a continuous light source that can be adjusted according to the patient's level of comfort and the photographer's ability to distinguish fine retinal detail. The viewing light is usually a tungsten bulb that is specific to a particular camera model. Changing the viewing lamp intensity does not affect the final fundus photograph.

A xenon-filled flash tube provides a brief burst of intense light that exposes the fundus photograph. The gas in the flash tube is ionized by the high voltage that is stored in the capacitors of the camera's power unit. Changing the intensity of the flash setting has no effect on the viewing illumination.

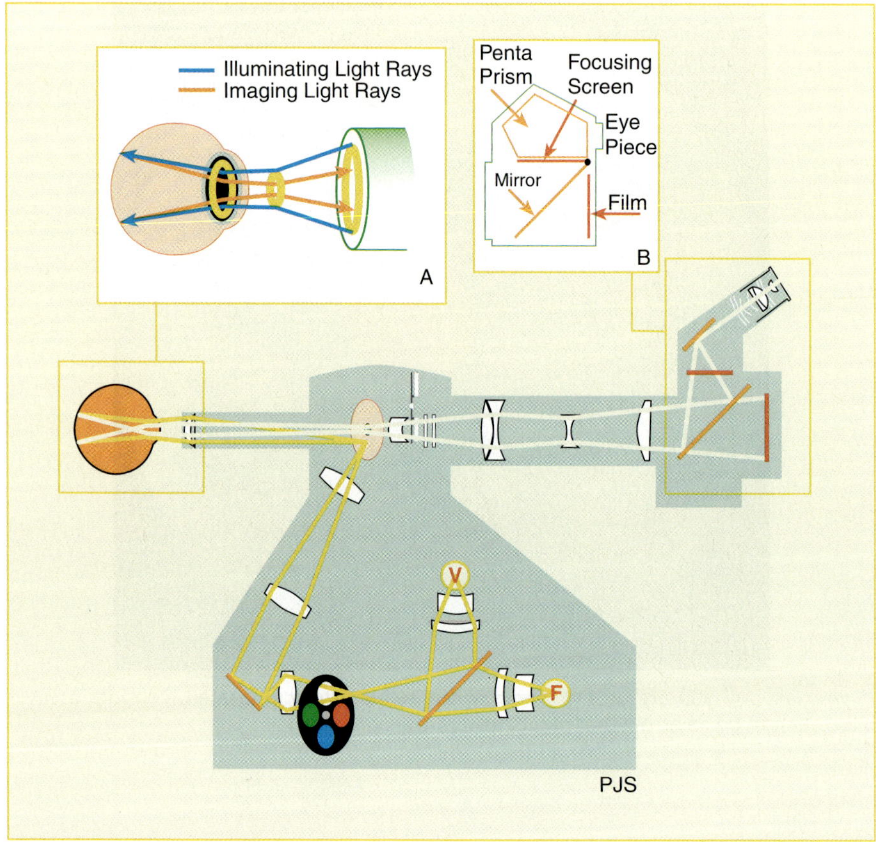

Figure 1–10 ○ The optical pathway of the fundus camera. Light generated from either the viewing lamp (V) or the electronic flash (F) is projected through a set of filters and onto a round mirror. The light reflects up into a series of lenses and exits the objective lens in the shape of a doughnut. Assuming that both the illumination system and the image are correctly aligned and focused, the resulting retinal image exits the cornea through the central, unilluminated portion of the doughnut (*inset A*). The light continues through the central aperture of the previously described mirror, through the astigmatic correction device and the diopter compensation lenses, and then back to the single lens reflex camera system (*inset B*).

Fundus cameras are often described by the angle of view—the optical angle of acceptance of the lens (Fig. 1–12). An angle of 30 degrees, considered the normal angle of view, creates a film image 2.5 times larger than life. Wide-angle fundus cameras image between 45 and 140 degrees and provide proportionately less retinal magnification. A narrow-angle fundus camera has an angle of view of 20 degrees or less. Normal-angle cameras have smaller illuminating annuli, making

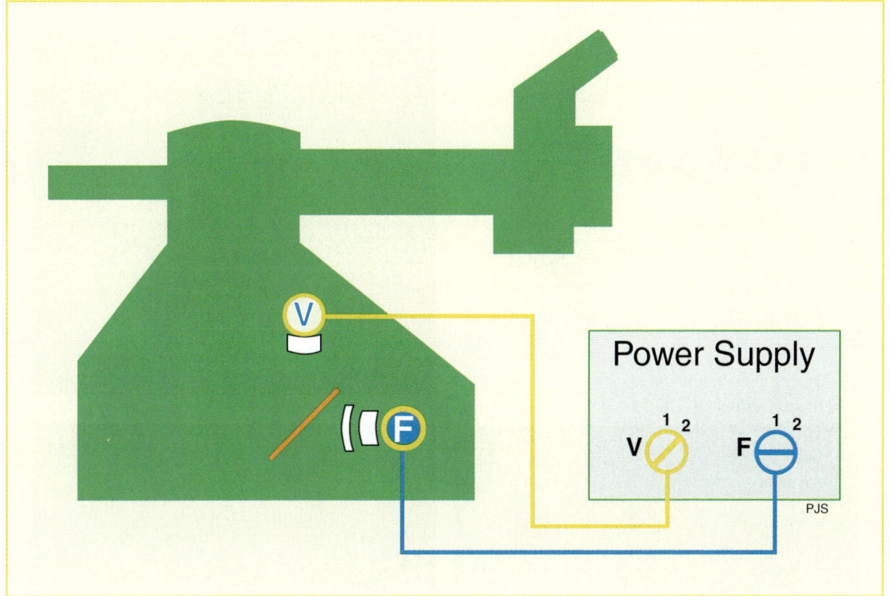

Figure 1–11 ○ The flash tube and the viewing lamp are controlled by separate electrical subsystems. Increase the flash setting if your pictures are too dark; increase the viewing lamp setting if your view of the fundus is dark.

them more suitable for patients with pupils of a smaller diameter. The inner diameter of the illuminating ring in wide-angle cameras is larger, making it more difficult to photograph patients with small pupils.

A number of specialized fundus camera designs exist. Extreme wide-angle cameras have an angle of acceptance of more than 150 degrees, usually contact the cornea during photography, and are useful when large retinal areas need to be documented (Fig. 1–13). Their small magnification minimizes fine retinal detail.

Simultaneous stereo fundus cameras use one exposure to place two images side by side on a single 35-mm frame (Fig. 1–14). Their standardized stereo base allows longitudinal studies of retinal topography as well as detailed electronic analysis of retinal topography.

Hand held fundus cameras provide maximum portability (Fig. 1–15). They are useful for photographing bedridden, infant, and animal patients.

Both mydriatic and nonmydriatic fundus cameras require patient dilation. Mydriatic fundus cameras require pharmacologic dilation, while nonmydriatic fundus cameras use infrared viewing systems to exploit the patient's natural dilation in a dark room. With nonmydriatic cameras, only a single image is captured, either digitally or on instant film. Nonmydriatic cameras are useful as documentation and screening devices.

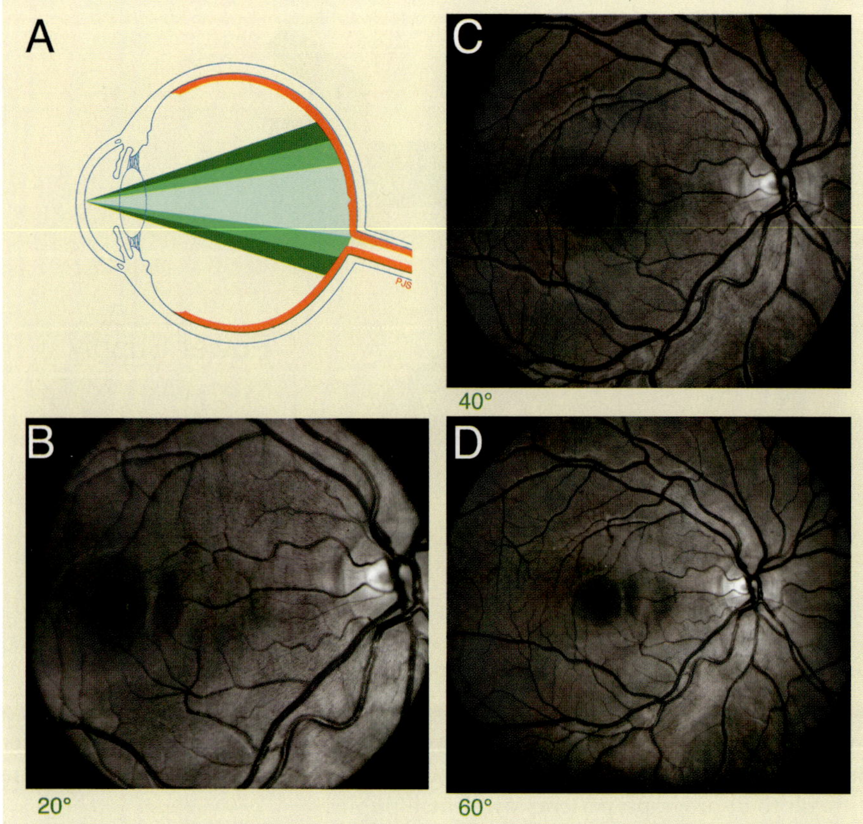

Figure 1–12 ○ Angles of view. The greater the angle of view, the larger the retinal area contained in the photograph (*A*). The smaller the angle of view, the greater the magnification. The same eye is photographed at 20 degrees (*B*), 40 degrees (*C*), and 60 degrees (*D*).

Nonmydriatic Fundus Cameras

The term *nonmydriatic fundus camera* is a bit of a misnomer. Mydriasis—widening of the pupil—is indeed required for this type of retinal photography. However, instead of pharmacologic dilation, the natural pupil dilation in a darkened room provides the window through which a patient's retina is photographed. Some users describe more consistent photographs when patients have been dilated with 1% mydriacyl.[13]

Infrared light (IR) is used to preview the retina on a video monitor. Once the monitor's image is focused and aligned, photographic technology takes over:

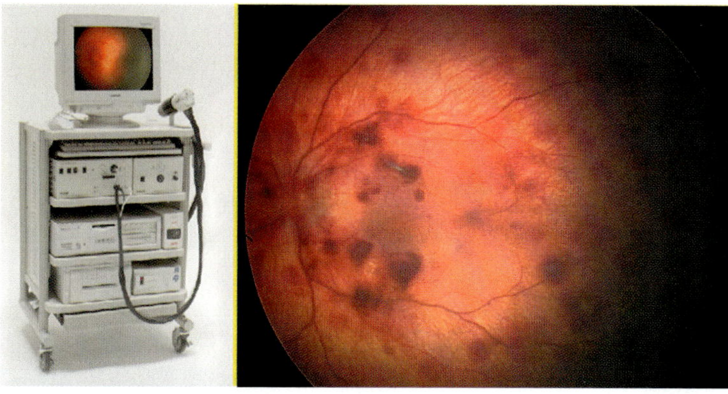

Figure 1–13 ○ The RetCam 120 (*left*) is a pediatric wide-angle contact lens camera. Its 120-degree angle of view captures the extent of hemorrhage in this patient with shaken baby syndrome (*right*). (Images courtesy Massie Research Laboratories, Inc. Dublin, CA, and Leslie D. MacKeen, CRA Hospital for Sick Children, Toronto, Canada.)

A flash is fired, and the image is exposed. The absence of a bright viewing/ alignment light can be a plus in pediatric fundus photography.

The nonmydriatic fundus camera was pioneered by Canon in the late 1970s, and by the mid-1980s, Canon, Kowa, Reichert, and Topcon were marketing various models. The typical angle of view of a nonmydriatic fundus camera is 45 degree. Many nonmydriatic cameras also feature a high magnification view for disc photography. While traditionally used for screening purposes, newer

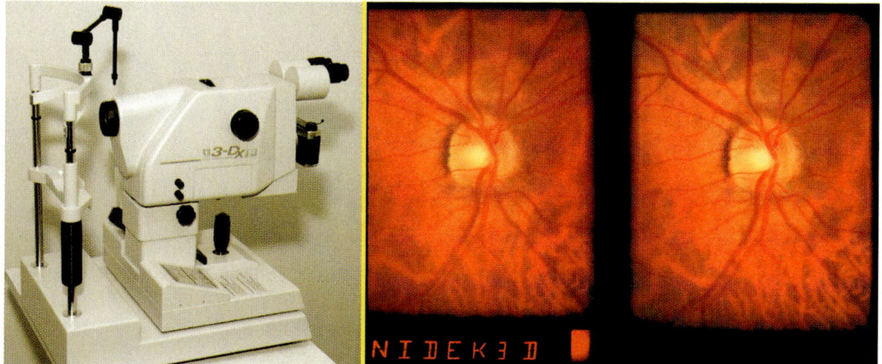

Figure 1–14 ○ The Nidek 3-Dx simultaneous stereo fundus camera (*left*) produces a side-by-side stereo pair on a single frame of 35-mm film (*right*).

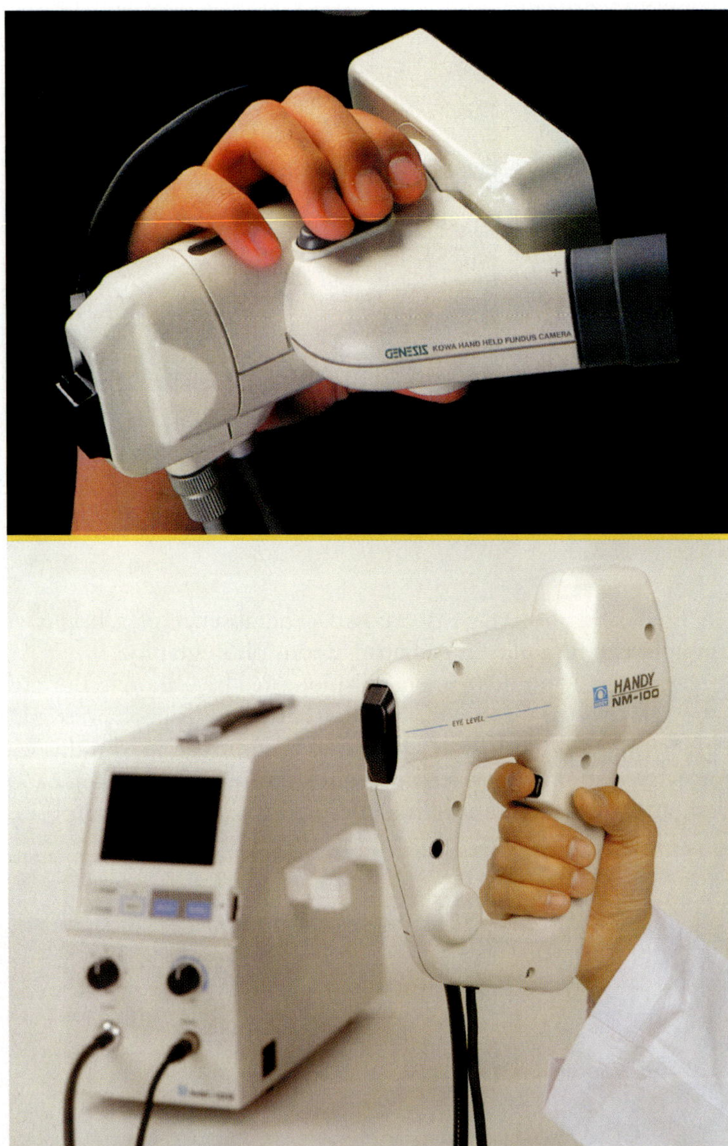

Figure 1–15 ○ Fundus photography of recumbent patients or animals is accomplished with a handheld fundus camera either on film using a Kowa Genesis (*top*) or digitally using a Nidek NM-100 (*bottom*). (Images courtesy of the manufacturers.)

"diabetic screening devices" substitute digitally databased electronic images for traditional Polaroid and 35-mm film.[14] The newest nonmydriatic fundus imaging technology is represented by the Optos (Fig. 1–16), a scanning laser ophthalmoscope that produces a 200-degree image.

Current "non-myds" use 1- to 3-MB digital chips to capture retinal images. Images are displayed on built-in LCD monitors and output to compact flash memory cards or a database via a USB connection. An advantage of these newer models is that their small chips function better in lower light levels than the traditional media, making the flash less bright and maximal dilation less of an issue—a plus for those whose primary imaging needs are for glaucoma patients.

You should not expect to perform stereo fundus photography or any type of ocular angiography with nonmydriatic cameras, as these techniques require multiple flashes. Because the flash can seem quite intense, warn the patient of afterimages. Since the alignment and focusing of these instruments differs from those of traditional fundus cameras, two sets of step-by-step instructions are included in the next chapter.

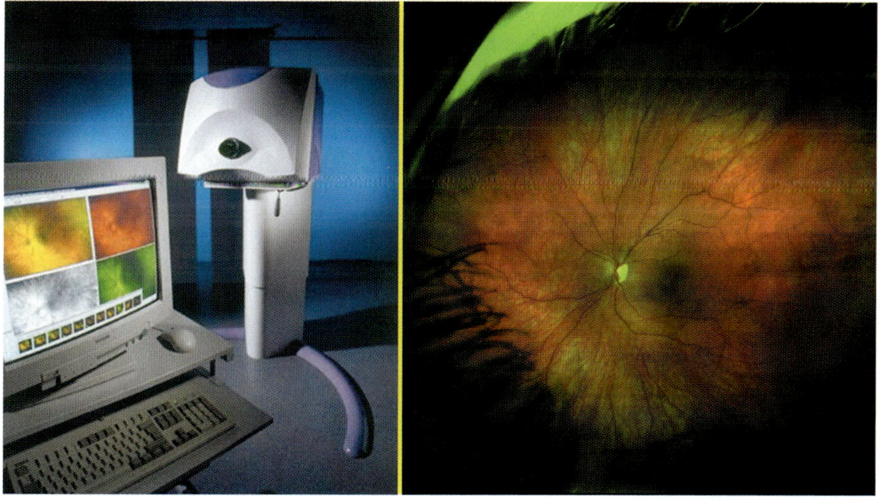

Figure 1–16 ○ The Optos Panoramic 200 Non-Mydriatic Ophthalmoscope (*left*) uses a scanning laser ophthalmoscope to produce a 200-degree image through an undilated pupil (*right*). (Images courtesy of Optos North America, Marlborough, MA.)

Selecting a Fundus Camera

Choosing a fundus camera is similar to buying an automobile. A family minivan is selected because of its versatility: It both transports people and hauls larger loads. It is not flashy or particularly fast, and it won't get the best gas mileage. A minivan is most like a medium-priced multiple-angle fundus camera. It offers respectable sharpness in a variety of optical angles and is suitable for a general ophthalmic practice.

A minivan won't outrace a sports car. Built for performance first and price second, the sports car is similar to the normal-angle fundus camera favored by the retinal specialist. It is designed to produce sharp photographs of the macula and does so extremely well. Its small illumination doughnut facilitates photographing through narrow pupils, and the astigmatic compensation device is useful for far peripheral views.

Special-use fundus cameras can be compared to pickup trucks or all-terrain vehicles. These include extreme wide-angle, simultaneous stereo, and hand-held fundus cameras. Minimal-feature, entry-level cameras and used models are inexpensive purchase options.

Pay careful attention to your specific needs when surveying the market. Compare and test-drive competing camera models during fundus photography workshops such as those sponsored by the Ophthalmic Photographers' Society. The FAQs on choosing a fundus camera found in Chapter 3 may help you prioritize fundus camera features and evaluate your needs.

Fundus Camera Controls

Each time you perform fundus photography, you will be adjusting a complex optical instrument in a darkened room filled with patients. Your mission: to completely familiarize yourself with each of your camera's controls. The alternative? Turning the light repeatedly on and off while you search for the appropriate setting, all the while cursing under your breath. Not a pretty picture.

Read your manual from cover to cover. Memorize it. If the manual is missing, contact the manufacturer to obtain another copy.

Figure 1–17 provides an overview of the controls found on most fundus cameras. Rely on your manual for the location and function of specific or specialized controls.

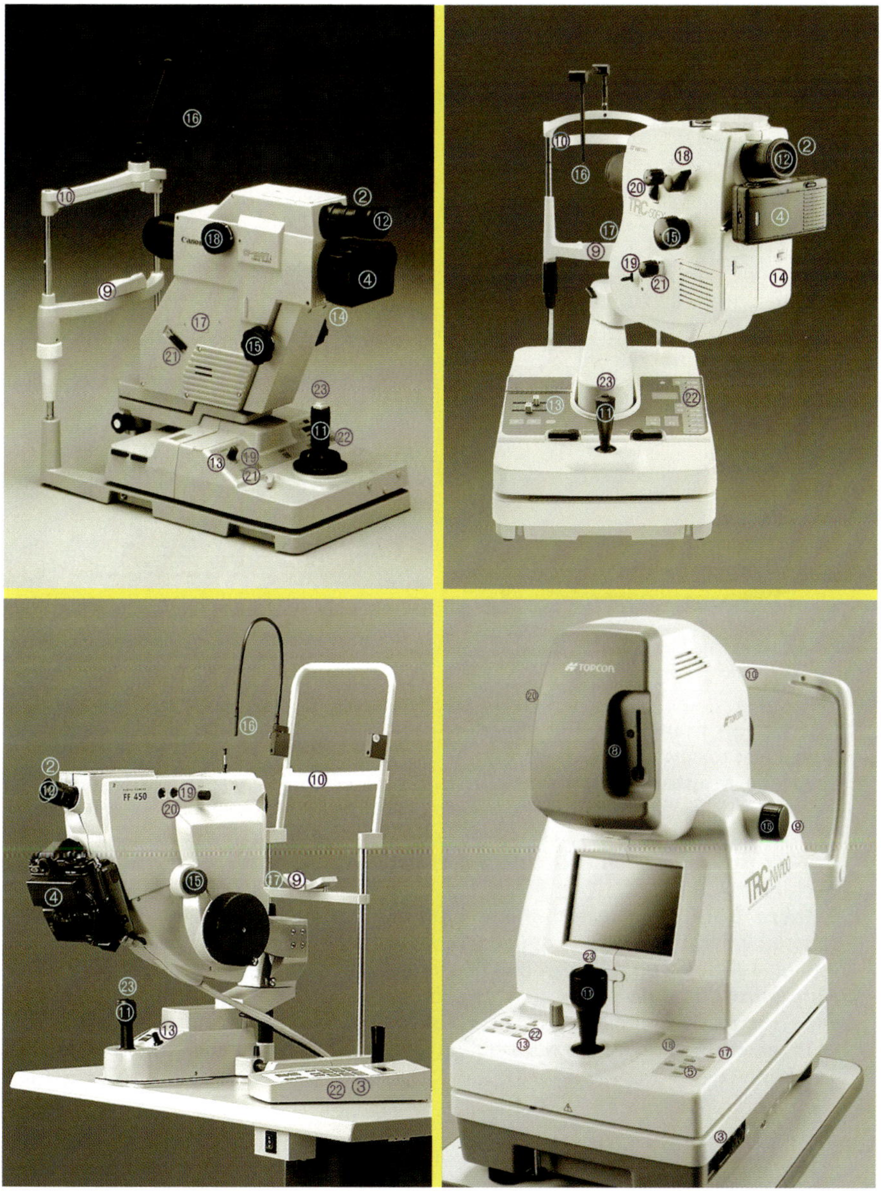

Figure 1–17 ○ In order of general usage, the controls of multiple fundus cameras are labeled to correspond to the following numbered descriptions. Your controls may vary according to the specific make and year of your fundus camera. (Images courtesy of Canon USA, Nidek, Topcon USA, and Humphrey Instruments/Carl Zeiss.)

(Figure continued on page 18)

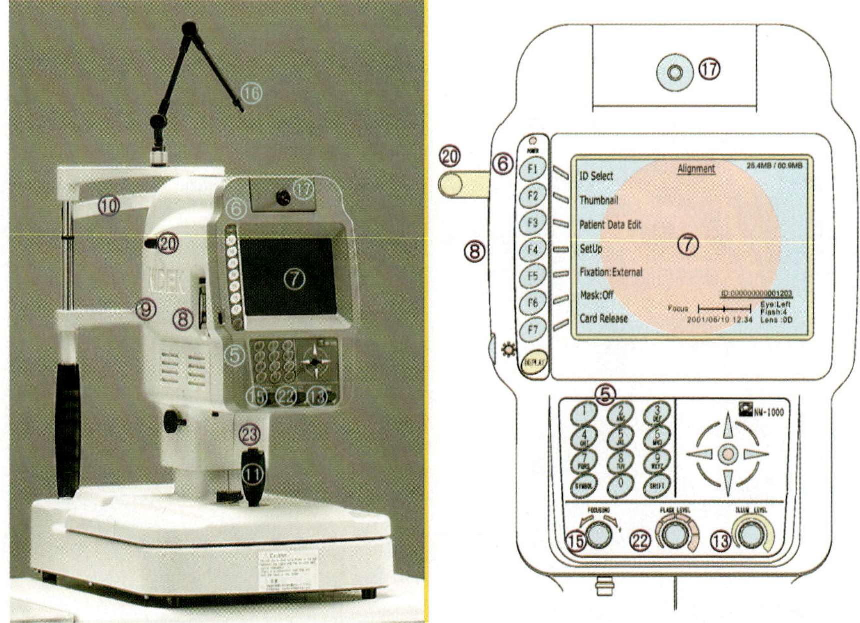

1. **Instruction manual.** Full of important information, this should be read studiously from cover to cover. (Not shown.)
2. **Eyepiece diopter adjustment.** Sets the eyepiece, allowing the photographer to view the reticle in sharp focus. The eyepiece must be correctly set, and the reticle must be in sharp focus to obtain sharp fundus photographs.
3. **On/off power switch.** Obvious, but essential—the master switch that controls all electrical functions.
4. **Camera back.** Traditionally, this is a light-tight container that holds film that is exposed when the shutter is opened. Modern fundus cameras offer a choice of conventional 35-mm film, video, instant film, or a digital chip. Make sure the film is loaded!
5. **Alphanumeric data entry.** Used to enter patient data onto a digital photograph.
6. **Function keys.** Context-specific keys that control standard settings.
7. **LCD screen.** To view the fundus during alignment using infrared and color images after capture.

8. **PC card slot.** Slot for inserting a Compact Flash Card.
9. **Chinrest.** Stabilizes the patient. This should be cleaned between patients.
10. **Forehead rest.** Stabilizes the patient. It should be cleaned immediately after patient contact.
11. **Joystick.** Controls the side-to-side and forward-to-backward motion of the optical head during photography.
12. **Ocular (eyepiece).** Allows you to view and judge the image before it is exposed. During fundus photography, keep both of your eyes open, relaxed, and focused on infinity.
13. **Viewing illumination control.** Adjusts the intensity of the viewing light. It has no effect on the brightness or darkness of the final fundus photograph.
14. **W.D.** Turns on and off the working distance dots: corneal reflections that help you align the fundus camera.
15. **Focusing knob.** Adjusts the distance between the front element and the focusing screen/film plane to maximize sharpness.
16. **External fixation light.** Used to direct patient fixation, this small light is universally positionable.
17. **Internal fixation device.** Small pointer that can be introduced into the optical pathway. It is useful for obtaining fixation in the eye you are photographing, for recording the retinal location of patient fixation, or as a pointer in a teaching slide. When not serving a specific purpose, it should be removed from the optical pathway before the picture is taken.
18. **Angle selection lever.** Inserts lenses into the optical pathway, which either increases or decreases the angle of view (or magnification). You should be familiar with the retinal area circumscribed by each setting, as well as the relative sharpness of each.
19. **Small pupil device.** Slightly decreases the diameter of the illumination ring on a wide-angle camera, improving photographs imaged through a smaller pupil. This device is usually ambitiously named; a single, normal-angle camera is the best choice in small pupil situations.
20. **Diopter compensation lens/anterior segment lens.** Places positive and/or negative lenses into the optical pathway, extending the focusing range to permit the photography of patients with unusually long or short eyes. The plus setting is used for external or anterior segment photographs.
21. **Filter insert/filter wheel.** Allows the addition of optional filters into the optical pathway, affecting the light that enters the eye.
22. **Flash intensity control.** Adjusts the amount of illumination emitted from the electronic flash. This control has no effect on the viewing illumination.
23. **Shutter release.** When pressed, exposes the photograph by initiating a series of events that includes raising the eyepiece mirror and opening the shutter, which triggers the flash.
24. **Lens cap.** Protects the front element. It should be placed over the lens whenever photographs are not being taken and immediately after each patient session. (Not shown.)

Fundus Camera Maintenance

Properly maintained, your fundus camera will provide years of reliable service. Surfaces that come into direct contact with the patient should be disinfected after each procedure and at the end of every day. Consult a member of your infection control team or your practitioner for currently recommended antimicrobial agents.

Keep two spare viewing lights, flash tubes, and fuses readily available. Know when and how to change them. Your fundus camera's instruction manual will contain detailed installation procedures. Alternatively, contact the manufacturer's technical representative.

The 35-mm camera body is the fundus camera's most frequently repaired component. Its shutter fires and its film transport gears rotate each time a photograph is exposed. Keep a spare camera body available.

You should be able to handle simple maintenance such as cleaning the front surface of the objective lens. Fundus cameras that are used daily should have yearly inspections by factory-trained technicians. Consider returning your camera to the factory for complete optical realignment and refurbishment every 5–10 years. Mobile cameras may need service more often.

References

1. Jackman WT, Webster JD: On photographing the retina of the living human eye. Philadelphia Photographer 1886;23:275.
2. Bedell AJ: Stereoscopic fundus photography. JAMA 1935;105:1502.
3. Dimmer F: Ueber die Photographie des Augenhintergrundes. Wiesbaden, Germany: Bergmann, 1907.
4. Dimmer F: Der Augenspiegel und die Ophthalmoskopische Diagnostik. Leipzig, Germany: F. Deuticke, 1921.
5. Dimmer F, Pillat A: Atlas photographischer Bilder des Menschlichen Augenhintergrundes. Leipzig, Germany: F. Deuticke, 1927.
6. Bedell AJ: Photographs of the Fundus Oculi. Philadelphia: F.A. Davis, 1929.
7. Edgerton HE: Photographic use of electrical discharge flashtubes. J Opt Soc Am 1946;36:390.
8. Rizzutti AB: High speed photography of the anterior ocular segment. Arch Ophthalmol 1950;43:365.
9. Ogle KN, Rucker CW: Fundus photographs in color using a high speed flash tube in the Zeiss retinal camera. Arch Ophthalmol 1953;49:435.
10. Hansell P, Beeson EJG: Retinal photography in color. Br J Ophthalmol 1953;37:65.
11. Parrish RK: The University of Miami Bascom Palmer Eye Institute Atlas of Ophthalmology. Boston: Butterworth-Heinemann, 2000.

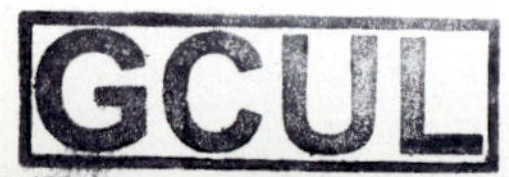

12. Harry J, Mission G: Clinical Ophthalmic Pathology. Boston: Butterworth-Heinemann, 2001.
13. Wade M, Barry C, McAllister I: Diabetic retinopathy screening in remote Australian communities with non-mydriatic fundus cameras. J Ophthalmol Photography 1998;20(3):80.
14. Bursell SE, Cavallerano JD, Cavallerano AA, et al.: Stereo nonmydriatic digital-video color retinal imaging compared with Early Treatment Diabetic Retinopathy Study seven standard field 35-mm stereo color photos for determining level of diabetic retinopathy. Ophthalmology 2001;108:572.

Chapter 2

Fundus Photography: Step by Step

Obtaining a good fundus photograph takes significantly longer than the tiny fraction of a second it takes to expose the film. As is true for the athlete who is judged on split-second decisions, proper preparation, standardized technique, and careful follow-through are vital to successful fundus photography. Read this chapter to learn a stepwise procedure (prepare, align, expose, and follow-up) for performing fundus photography with either a mydriatic (below) or a nonmydriatic (page 35) camera.

Fundus Photography with a Mydriatic Camera

Most fundus cameras are mydriatic fundus cameras. The patient's eyes must be pharmacologically dilated prior to fundus photography with a mydriatic camera. Follow the steps below for successful fundus photography (Table 2–1).

Prepare

1. **Prepare the room.** The room should be clean and tidy, and the camera should be disinfected between patients. All billing, tracking, and other paperwork should be completed before the patient is escorted to the camera. Select the appropriate camera back, and load it with a color slide film.
2. **Adjust the eyepiece.** Set your reticle (see the accompanying box on page 25). Photograph a name tag before the patient enters the room to reassure yourself that the camera is functioning properly and to serve as a guidepost during editing. You won't be looking into the eyepiece again until Step 9.
3. **Plan the photographs.** Take a moment to prepare yourself for the procedure. Review the photo request form (Fig. 2–1). Examine prior photographs.

Table 2–1
Fundus Photography: Step by Step

Prepare	Prepare the room
	Adjust the eyepiece
	Plan the photographs
	Escort your patient
	Inform your patient
	Position your patient
	Position yourself
Align	Establish fixation
	Position the illumination system
	Adjust the joystick
	Select the area of interest
	Select the angle of view
	Check the focus
Expose	Double-check everything
	Expose the film
	Close the session
Follow-up	Process your film
	Review your work
	Edit and label your photographs
	Deliver the finished product

Note: Review these steps before or during the procedure to help establish your routine. Post a copy of these steps near your fundus camera for reference.

Note the patient's visual acuity and working diagnosis. Have a photographic plan in mind that includes your angle of view selections, the areas of the patient's retina you intend to document, and any specialized techniques that may be useful.

4. **Escort your patient.** Check that your patient's pupils are fully dilated. Your demeanor should be bright but professional. Offer to take a coat or other personal items, setting them on the available shelf or hook. Invite your patients to be seated, and introduce yourself with a smile. Talk to your patients throughout the procedure; reassure them and let them know what to expect.

5. **Inform your patient.** Informed patients are cooperative patients. Ask your patients whether they have had their eyes photographed before. Explain the procedure, acquainting them with the impending bright flashes and with your expectations. Let them know that it is fine for them to blink and breathe normally. Reassure them that the multicolored spots they will see afterward are nothing to worry about. Tell them that it is just like looking into a flash when they are having their picture taken and that no X-rays are involved.

Setting Your Reticle

To obtain a sharp view of the reticle, your eyepiece must be correctly set. Here is a step-by-step procedure for eyepiece adjustment:

1. **Have your eyes corrected for their best visual acuity.** *You may choose to photograph with or without glasses or contact lenses if your correction is spherical. Remember, however, that the correct eyepiece setting will be different depending on whether you wear your corrective lenses. If you have astigmatism, you should wear your corrective lenses while adjusting the eyepiece. Do not wear reading glasses.*

2. **Eliminate any subject matter from the camera's field of view.** *Set your camera to the farthest focusing extreme, and hold or tape a piece of white cardboard in front of the objective lens. When you look through the viewfinder, you should see a blurry reticle on a white field. The illumination level should be adjusted to a medium or low setting (approximately the same intensity as when viewing the retina). If the picture is too bright, it may cause your pupil to constrict, bringing depth of field into play and making an accurate setting difficult.*

3. **Set the eyepiece adjustment to the maximum plus diopter setting.** *This will blur any image of the focusing reticle. When looking through the viewfinder, you should see an evenly illuminated white field.*

4. **Relax your eyes.** *Blink and look at something far away—perhaps down a long hall or at a reflection. It is extremely important that your eyes be focused on infinity to obtain the correct setting. Keeping both eyes open may help to keep you from accommodating.*

5. **Peer through the viewfinder, and begin turning the eyepiece ring toward the zero setting.** *Smoothly rotate the ring. Rotate at a slow enough rate that you perceive the reticle becoming sharper but not so slowly that your eyes accommodate for the change. Remember to keep both eyes open and focused at infinity.*

6. **Stop rotating when the reticle is just in sharp focus.** *If you continue to rotate the reticle after you achieve sharp focus, or if you begin to search for sharpness by rotating the reticle back and forth, then accommodation may be influencing your decision. If your eyes are at their best correction, your setting will probably be within a diopter or so of the zero mark. If your diopter setting is a high minus, chances are that you have accommodated. If you are wearing no correction, the setting should be within a diopter of your best correction.*

7. **Repeat, repeat, repeat.** *Continue setting the eyepiece until three successive near-normal settings agree. Note the most consistent position of the eyepiece ring. Remember to set the eyepiece correctly before each patient session. New photographers should repeat this exercise daily until they are confident that their eyepiece setting is accurate.*

   Each fundus camera should be set individually by each photographer. The correct setting for each camera (especially if brands vary) may be slightly different for the same photographer, and the correct setting for a single camera will vary between photographers in the same office. If an instrument has more than one user, a signal can be developed to alert alternate users of possible eyepiece setting changes (perhaps an empty film box placed over the eyepiece).

8. **Check the eyepiece setting and reticle before each patient.** *It cannot be overemphasized that once your personal setting has been ascertained, it is imperative to check it before each patient. Be aware of the focusing screen's reticle throughout each photographic procedure.* Only conscientious use of the eyepiece/reticle focusing system will ensure consistently sharp fundus photographs.

Dartmouth-Hitchcock Medical Center
OPHTHALMIC PHOTOGRAPHY REQUEST FORM
Posterior Segment

Date _________　Physician ___________

V　Hx/Dx:________________________
　　　________________________
　　　________________________
Signature ____________________

Fundus Photography

OD　　OS

1　Disc　1
2　Macula　2
3　　3
4　　4
5　　5
6　　6
7　　7

Field 8
(please sketch)

PJS

OTHER:
☐　Wide angle　☐　Red Filt.　☐　Kowa Handheld
☐　High mag　☐　Green Filt.　☐　Torsion
☐　SL Fundus　☐　Blue Filt.

Angiography

☐ **Fluorescein**
☐ ICG

☐　Patient wait
☐　Patient go
☐　Call
☐　No Call

LOCATION ☐　**Disc** ☐　**Mac.** ☐　**Other** (above)

TRANSIT　　☐ **OD**　☐ **OS**
LATES　☐ **OU** ☐ **OD**　☐ **OS** ☐ **Scan**

INJECTION

☐　500mg 10% NaFl injected by ____________

☐　50mg ICG injected by ____________

INTERPRETATION & REPORT

PHOTOGRAPHER 'S NOTE:

Media: ☐　Clear
　　☐ Hazy
　　☐ Poor

Coop: ☐　Good
　　☐ Fair
MD SIGNATURE __________ ☐ Poor

Consent for Angiography　　Date___________

I hereby authorize employees of DHMC to inter-view me, photograph, or otherwise illustrate portions of my anatomy. I further agree that they may use , and permit others persons to use information, slides, negatives, prints and other video or audio recordings for medical, scientific, educational or other related purposes.

I hereby authorize employees of DHMC to adminis-ter intravenous angiography. I have been informed of the nature and purpose of the procedure, as well as risks and possible side effects. I understand the available alternatives including the risks, conse-quences, and probable effectiveness of each. Likewise, I am aware of the prognosis and possible consequences if the procedure is not performed.

Signed
____

Witness
____

Routing:　White - Eye Chart　Yellow - Medical Records　Rev 12/97 C-358A

Figure 2–1 ○ Photography request form. Using a photography request form facilitates communication between the practitioner and the photographer. One form should be completed for each patient photography session.

6. **Position your patient.** Comfortable patients are cooperative patients. Adjust the patient's chair height, then the height of the camera, and finally the height of your chair (Fig. 2–2). Instruct the patient to place his or her chin in the chinrest and forehead against the bar. Raise or lower the table height or adjust the chinrest as needed. When correctly positioned at the fundus camera, your patient should have a straight back and be leaning slightly forward. The height of his or her eyes should approximately correspond to the height of the objective lens. Glasses should be off, but nontinted contact lenses may be in.

7. **Position yourself.** After the patient has been made comfortable, you should do likewise. Your eye should be at the same height as the viewfinder; raise or lower your seat as appropriate. A typist uses the "home row" to standardize

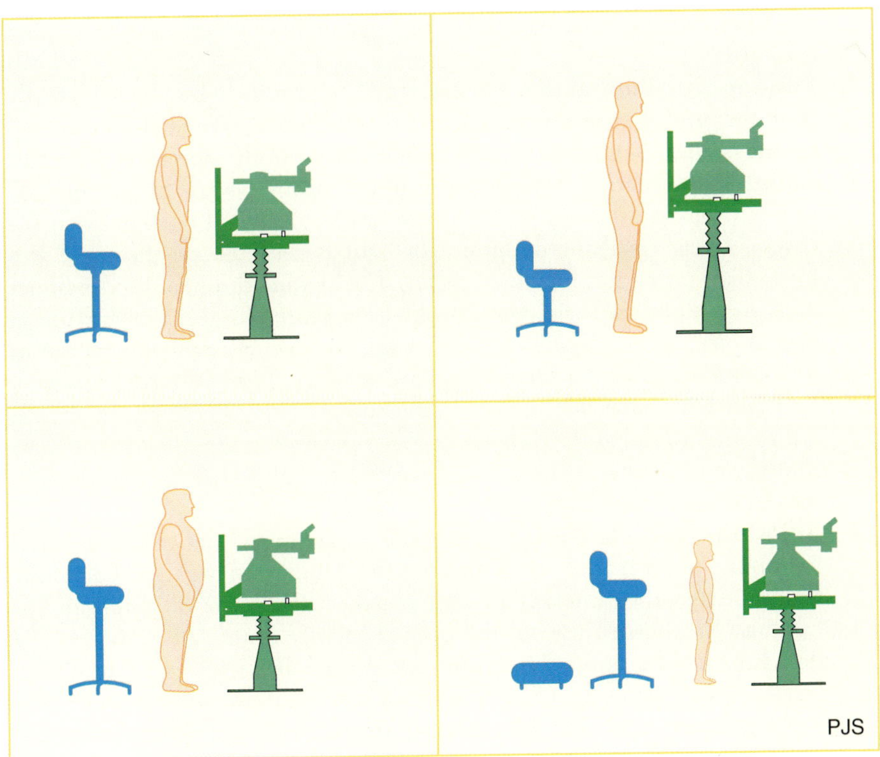

Figure 2–2 ○ Seating the patient. Both the chair and the camera are adjusted to their midpoint for the average-sized patient (*top left*). Lower the chair and raise the camera for tall or long-bodied patients (*top right*). Raise the chair and lower the camera for heavy or short patients (*bottom left*). A child's height will dictate the best seating strategy. The child may be comfortable while standing flat on the floor or on a short step stool (*bottom right*).

interaction with the keyboard. In the same way, you are encouraged to find your own "home keys." Grip the joystick with your dominant hand. If the optical head height adjustment is a separate control, place your other hand on it, extending it upward for the focusing knob or external fixation device. The index finger of the joystick hand or the right foot triggers the shutter release. Use the hand closest to the power supply for adjustments there.

Align

8. **Establish fixation.** Ask the patient to look straight ahead. Slide the fundus camera in front of the eye to be photographed. A fixation target is much more useful for fundus photography than it is during a slit lamp exam. Present the external fixation light to the eye that is not being photographed, and ask the patient to keep looking at it. Let the patient know that the small light will be in the middle of the bigger light once you have everything centered.

9. **Position the illumination system.** Turn the room lights down. Grossly align the fundus camera from side to side until the viewing light is centered on the cornea. Keep the joystick upright, and use the optical head height adjustment as needed. Position the illumination system by moving the forehead rest adjustment (or camera or patient) toward or away from the objective lens until the doughnut of light is centered on the pupil and focused on the cornea (or closed eyelid). On looking through the viewfinder with your dominant eye, you should see a blurry fundus image with an overlapping reticle (Fig. 2–3). The image you see will probably be out of focus and may have a crescent-shaped artifact. Focus quickly, knowing that you will make fine focusing adjustments later. The crescent-shaped artifact indicates that the distance between the objective lens and the cornea is nearly correct. An unsharp or fuzzy artifact implies that the illumination system is improperly aligned.

10. **Adjust the joystick.** The location of the crescent indicates your centration within the pupil (Fig. 2–4). If the crescent is found on the right side of the fundus image, the camera is off-center to the right side of the pupil. In this case, use the joystick to shift the camera slightly to the left, centering the doughnut in the pupil. These crescent-shaped artifacts can occur above, below, and to each side. Using the joystick, move in the direction opposite to the crescent to recenter the camera in the pupil and eliminate the artifact. Once your view is free of crescent-shaped artifacts, seek proper color saturation. Moving the joystick toward and away from the patient, check for the most even, most fully saturated view.

11. **Select the area of interest.** Your photographic plan (Step 3) should specify the areas you intend to photograph. If no posterior pole photographs

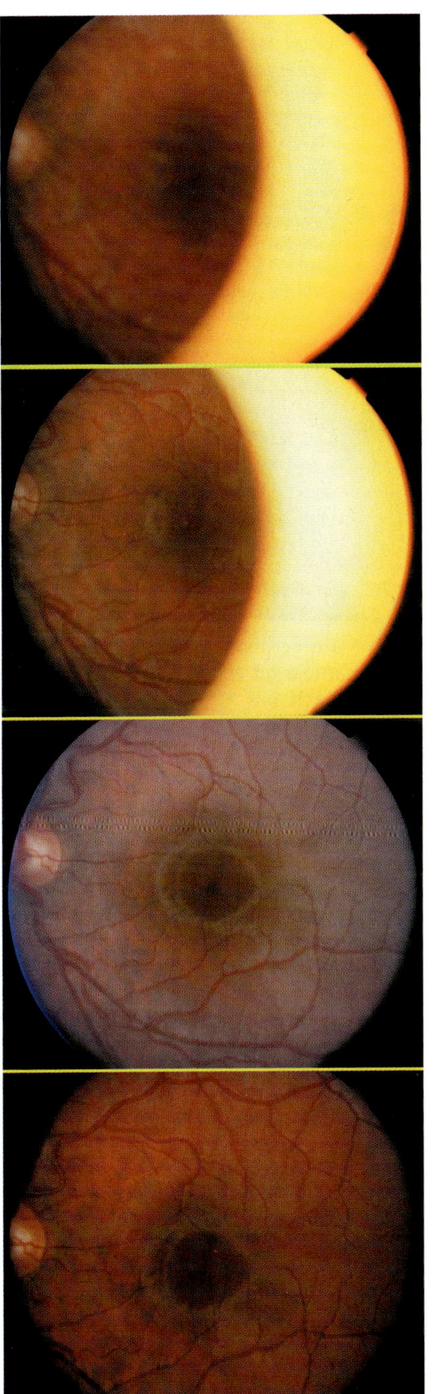

Figure 2–3 ○ Just after you align the optical system, your look through the viewfinder will probably look blurry and contain artifacts (*top*). After a quick focus (*second*), move up and down or from side to side to eliminate all crescent artifacts (*third*), then move forward and backward to find the maximum color saturation (*bottom*). Finally, focus carefully on the retinal details.

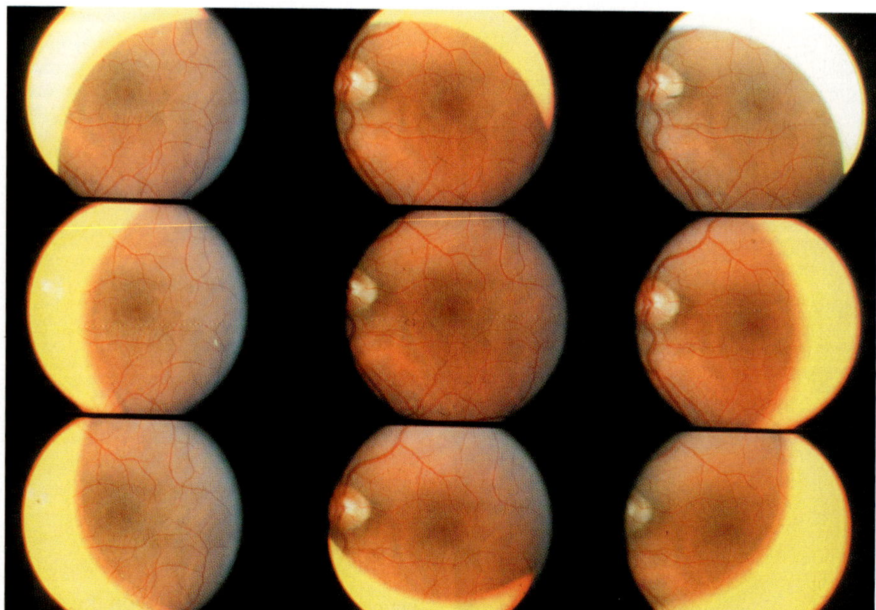

Figure 2–4 ○ Centering the camera. When the camera is centered on the pupil (*center*), you will see no position-related artifacts. Moving the camera off-center causes a reflection from the edge of the dilated pupil. This happens along each axis.

have been requested, it is a good idea to photograph the macula of each eye first to ensure a familiar landmark during the editing process. Adjust the external fixation device until the area of interest is centered in the field of view.

12. **Select the angle of view.** Your choice of magnification depends on both the patient and the characteristics of the pathology. A normal or narrow angle of view is used to document fine retinal details (Fig. 2–5). Recording the extent of a retinal condition requires a wide angle of view (Fig. 2–6). Consider using multiple angles of view (Fig. 2–7): Fundus photographs depicting the extent of a vein occlusion may benefit from a wide angle of view, whereas photographs of macular edema in the same eye should be made using a narrower angle of view.

13. **Check the focus.** Look critically at the reticle and the fundus image. Ask your patient to blink if he or she is not doing so naturally. Begin turning the focusing knob, and the retinal image will sharpen. While remaining aware of the focusing reticle, keep turning the knob, and the major blood vessels will become sharp. Concentrate on the next smaller blood vessel

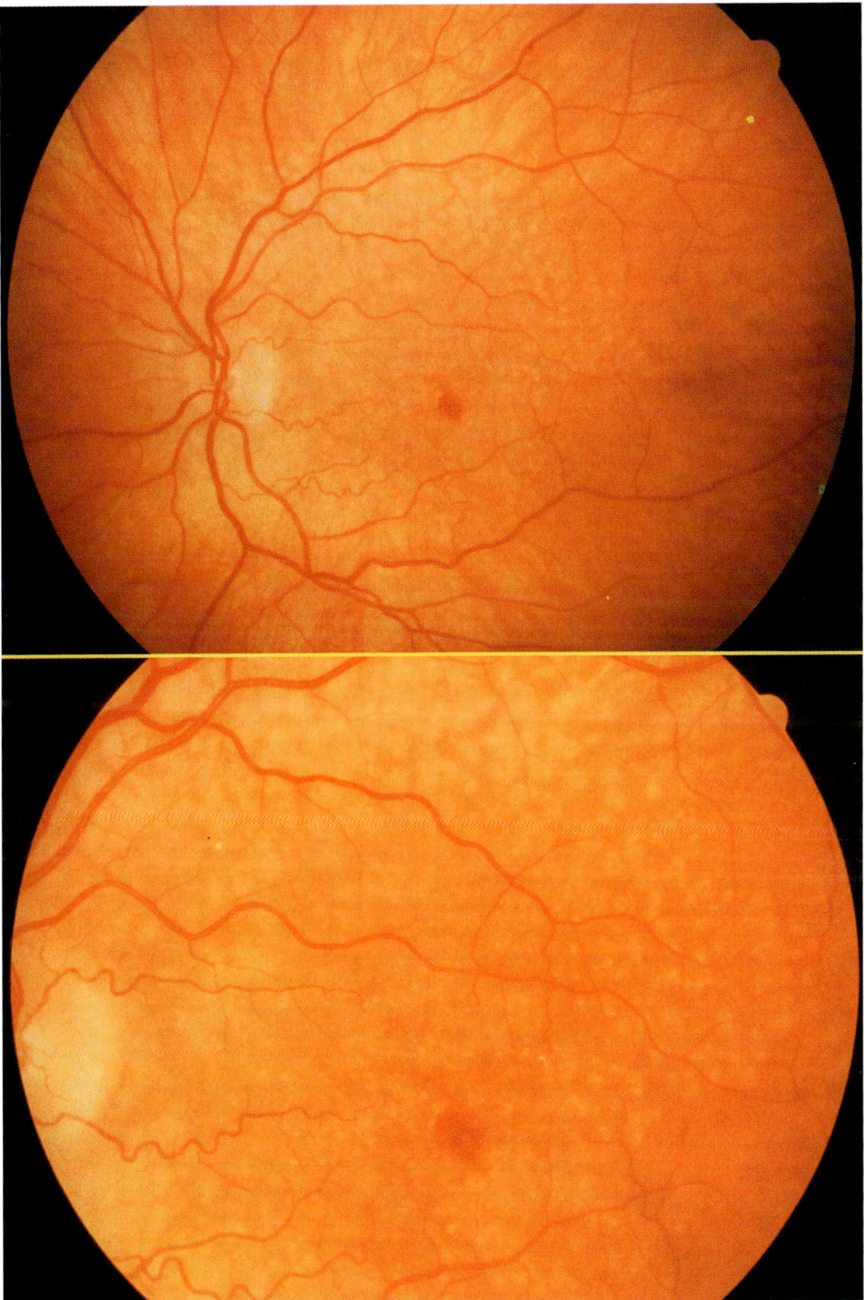

Figure 2–5 ○ Normal- or narrow-angle fundus photographs are used to document fine retinal details. More macular detail is revealed by the 30-degree photograph (*bottom*) than by the 60-degree photograph (*top*).

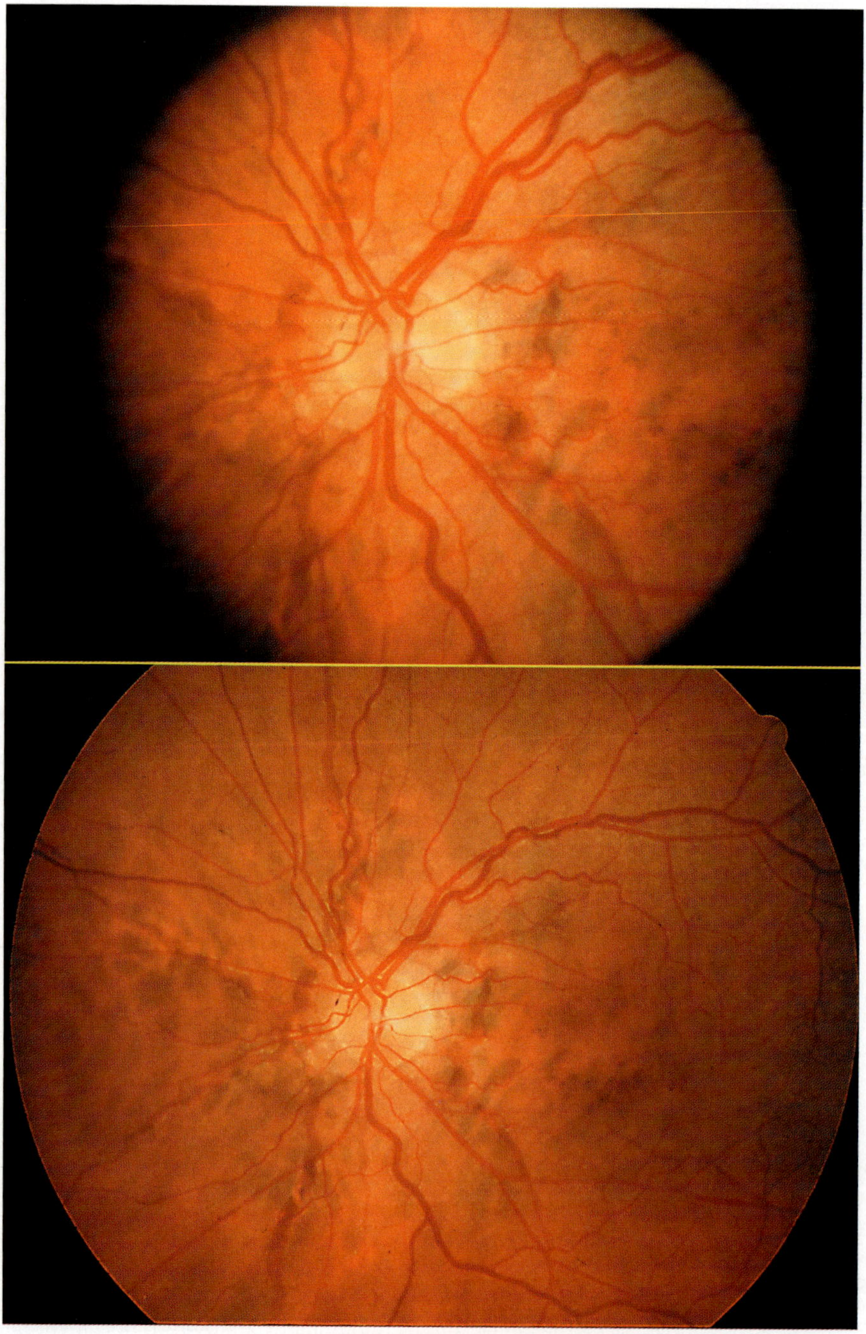

Figure 2–6 ○ Wide-angle fundus photographs are used to document the extent of a retinal condition. While the normal-angle photograph reveals fine detail of the optic nerve (*top*), the 60-degree photograph (*bottom*) better documents the extent of the angioid streaks.

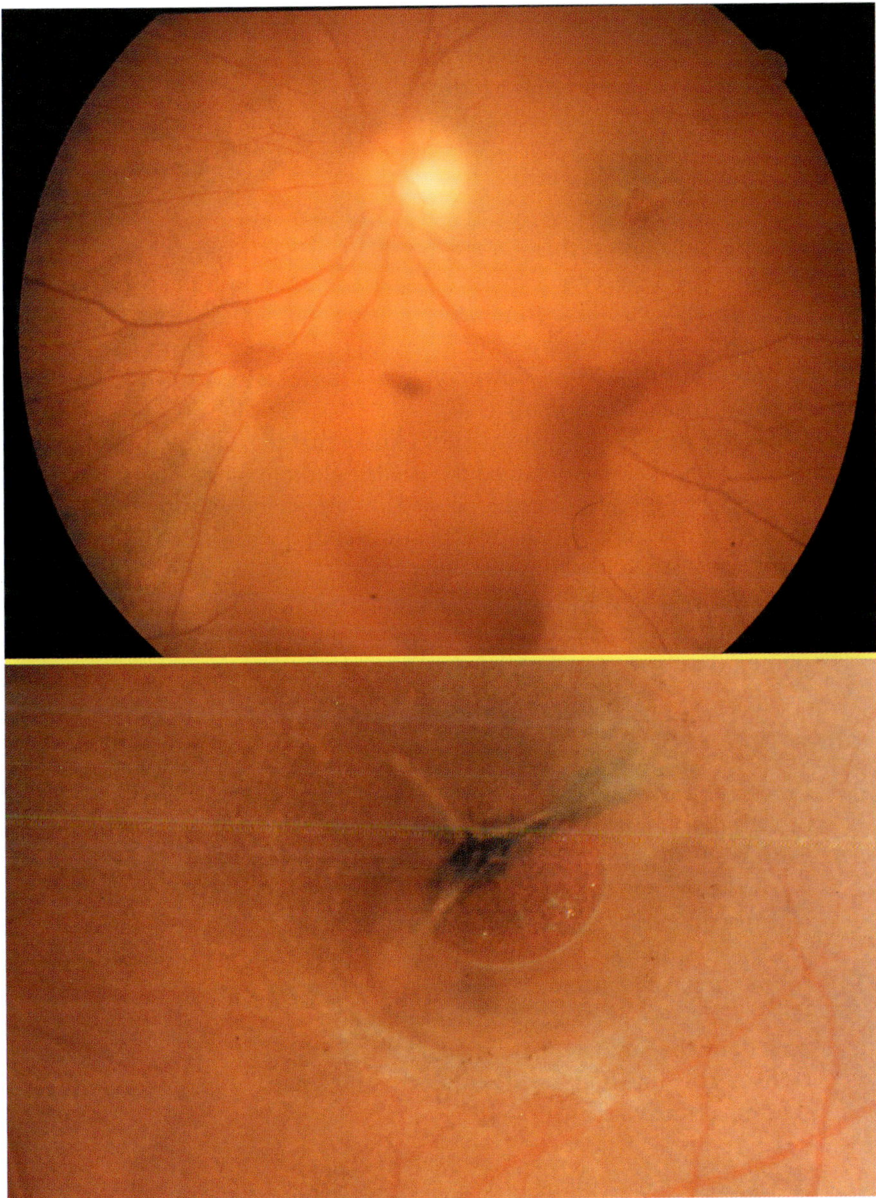

Figure 2–7 ○ Consider using multiple angles of view in the same patient. Combining a wide-angle view (*top*) with a narrow-angle view (*bottom*) is effective in showing the retinal damage from this industrial laser accident.

branches and then the next smaller branches. In very clear eyes, you may be able to distinguish extremely fine blood vessels. Eyes with cataracts or other media opacities may reveal only the major blood vessels. Focus as best as you can, remembering that not every patient has clear media.

Expose

14. **Double-check everything.** Develop the habit of quickly reviewing major variables just before the exposure. Make sure that both the reticle and the retina are in focus. Fine-tune your focusing and field of view. Monitor the image for maximum color saturation and the absence of artifacts.
15. **Expose the film.** Press down on the shutter release button to take a picture. (It's as easy as that!)
16. **Close the session.** Let your patients know that they did well (even if they did not) and that you obtained the needed photographs (which you should have). Remind them that the colors they are seeing are normal. Reassure them that the spots will go away soon. Remind them that fundus photography is just like looking into a flash when they get their picture taken. Release the patient with a smile, making sure that he or she feels fine and knows where the next clinic stop is. Complete all paperwork, including signing the chart.

Follow-Up

17. **Process your film.** Have your color film promptly developed by a professional processing laboratory.
18. **Edit, label, and review your photographs.** Edit the film promptly after it is returned from the processor; keep the best images and discard the rest. Label each slide with the patient's number, the date taken, the referring practitioner, and the patient's diagnosis. Always take some time during the editing process to examine your work with an eye toward quality control. How could this photograph have been more effective? What could have been done to eliminate that artifact?
19. **Deliver the finished product.** Insert the patient's photographs in the chart in a timely manner.

Fundus Photography with a Nonmydriatic Camera

Follow the steps below for successful nonmydriatic fundus photography (Table 2–2).

Table 2–2 **Nonmydriatic Fundus Photography: Step by Step**	
Prepare	Prepare the room Plan the photographs Escort your patient Inform your patient Position your patient Position yourself
Align	External alignment View the fundus Establish fixation Focus the image Adjust the joystick
Expose	Double-check everything Coach the patient Expose the image Photograph the other eye Close the session
Follow-up	Label/archive your photographs Deliver the finished product Review your work

Note: Review these steps before or during the procedure to help establish your routine. Post a copy of these steps near your nonmydriatic fundus camera for reference.

Prepare

1. **Prepare the room.** The room should be clean and tidy; the camera should be disinfected between patients. All billing, tracking, and other paperwork should be completed before the patient is escorted to the camera. Turn the camera on, enter the patient information, and insert the compact flash card (digital) or make sure film is loaded (film).

2. **Plan the photographs.** Take a moment to prepare yourself for the procedure. Review the photo request form (see Fig. 2–1). Examine prior photographs. Note the patient's visual acuity and working diagnosis. Have a photographic plan in mind that includes your angle of view selections, the areas of the patient's retina you intend to document, and any specialized techniques that may be useful.

3. **Escort your patient.** Your demeanor should be bright but professional. Talk to your patients throughout the procedure; reassure them and let them know what to expect.

4. **Inform your patient.** Informed patients are cooperative patients. Ask your patients whether they have had their eyes photographed before. Explain the

procedure, acquainting them with the impending bright flashes and with your expectations. Let them know that it is fine for them to blink and breathe normally. Reassure them that the multicolored spots they will see afterward are nothing to worry about. Tell them that it is just like looking into a flash when they are having their picture taken and that no X-rays are involved.

5. **Position your patient.** Comfortable patients are cooperative patients. Adjust the patient's chair height, then the height of the camera, and finally the height of your chair (see Fig. 2–2). Instruct the patient to place his or her chin in the chinrest and forehead against the bar. Raise or lower the table height or adjust the chinrest as needed. When correctly positioned at the fundus camera, your patient should have a straight back and be leaning slightly forward. The height of his or her eyes should approximately correspond to the height of the objective lens. Glasses should be off, but nontinted contact lenses may be in.

6. **Position yourself.** After the patient has been made comfortable, you should do likewise. A typist uses the "home row" to standardize interaction with the keyboard. In the same way, you are encouraged to find your own "home keys." Grip the joystick with your dominant hand. If the optical head height adjustment is a separate control, place your other hand on it, extending it upward for the focusing knob or external fixation device. The index finger of the joystick hand or the right foot triggers the shutter release. Use the hand closest to the power supply for adjustments there.

Align

7. **External alignment.** Viewing the patient's external eye as an IR image on the monitor, align by centering the "W.D." (working distance alignment dots) on the pupil (Fig. 2–8). Depending on the particular model of camera, two or three bright dots or a vertical light beam will reflect off of the cornea to help you judge the extent of dilation. If the patient's pupil is not larger than the area outlined by these corneal reflectors, the pupil may be too small for successful nonmydriatic photography. More time (2–3 minutes) and a darker room may improve natural dilation, or you may need to instill dilating drops.

8. **View the fundus.** To see the patient's fundus, you will likely move the camera straight toward the pupil (you may need to rotate the internal view knob). Adjust the illumination intensity control for your best view. As long as the infrared filter is in place, the patient should not react to changes in illumination.

9. **Establish fixation.** Ask the patient to look straight ahead. Most nonmydriatic cameras present a choice of internal fixation targets: commonly a centered stick with a split-image focusing light, and a blinking light on the temporal

side. The central internal fixation target will help you achieve a well-centered photograph of the macula, while the off-center internal fixation light will provide a posterior pole or disc photograph, depending on the chosen magnification.

10. **Focus the image.** The image you see on the monitor will probably be out of focus and may have a crescent-shaped artifact or fuzzy edges. Focus using the split-image range finder: Align the central lights until they form one single bar, adjusting the illumination as needed (Fig. 2–9).

If the patient is heavily myopic or hyperopic, you might need to use the diopter compensation lens selector. Use the "plus" for short eyes and the "minus" for long eyes and external (iris) views. The effect will be immediately seen on the infrared video monitor (the split-image focusing mechanism might not be active).

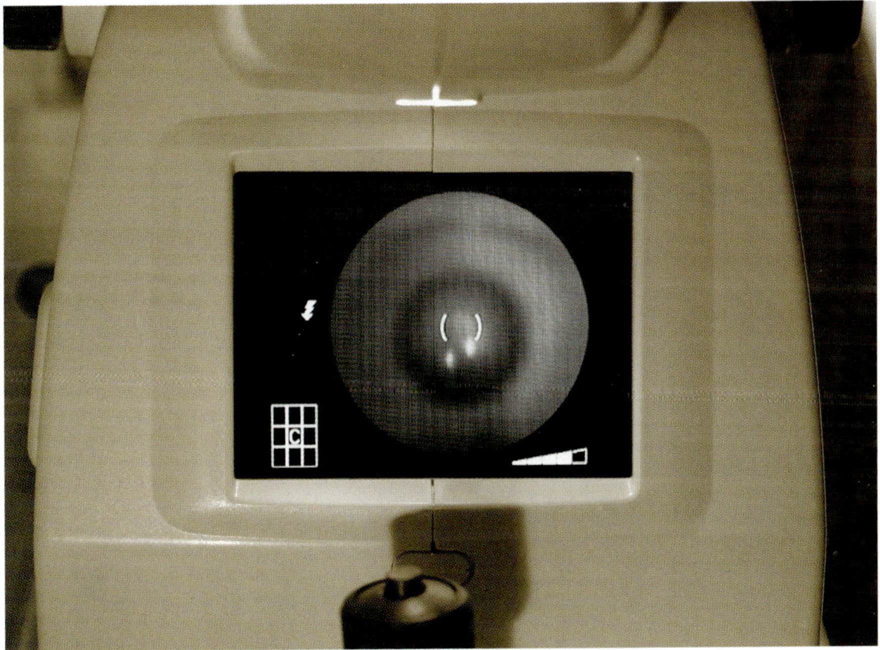

Figure 2–8 ○ Align the camera externally first. As you move the instrument closer to the patient using the joystick, bring the two bright working distance spots together to form a single spot within the brackets. This screen view of a Topcon NW6S indicates the infrared illumination level (*lower right*) and that the flash has recycled (*lightning bolt on left*). The nine-square matrix represents the internal fixation points. The Mosaic feature of this camera will digitally stitch together multiple images to create a wide field view. A blinking "C" in the central box alerts the user that the central field of the Mosaic feature has been selected. (Images courtesy Gary S. Michalec, CRA, Veterans Administration Medical Center, Minneapolis, MN.)

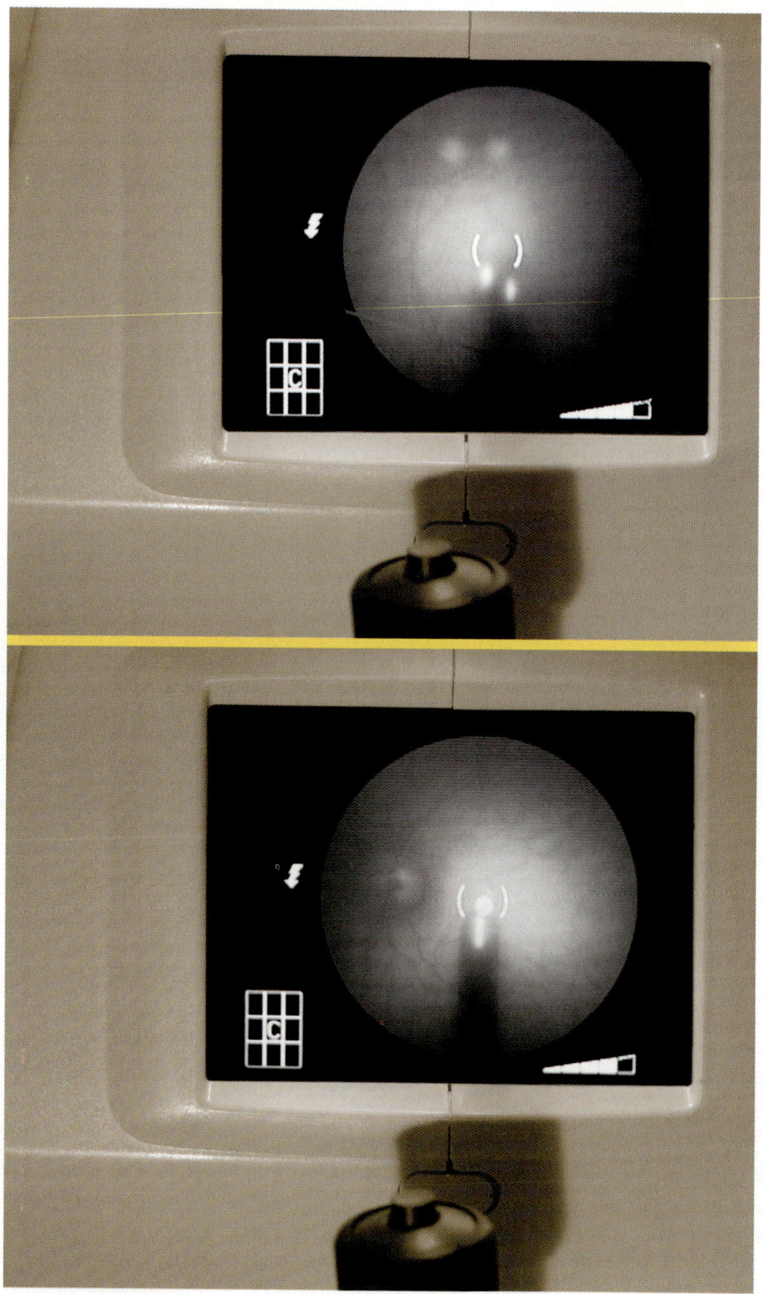

Figure 2–9 ○ Focus the image by rotating the focusing knob until the broken lines of the split-image rangefinder become a single line. It can be difficult to accurately evaluate the clarity of focus in an infrared image. Have the patient blink, check the fixation, and encourage the patient to open his or her eyes wide just before you press the shutter. (Images courtesy Gary S. Michalec, CRA, Veterans Administration Medical Center, Minneapolis, MN.)

11. **Adjust the joystick.** Look for two or three working distance corneal reflections and use the joystick to align the camera so that either the multiple reflections merge in the center to become a single reflection or two sharp, round reflections are seen at 9:00 and 3:00.

    You might see crescent-shaped artifacts on the periphery of your image. If the crescent is found on the right side of the fundus image, the camera is off-center to the right side of the pupil. Using the joystick, move in the opposite direction of the crescent to recenter the camera in the pupil (and eliminate the artifact). Look around the periphery of the image; if the edge of the image is cloudy or blurry, either adjust the joystick toward or away from the patient until the whole image is clear, ask the patient to blink twice, or ask the patient to open his or her eyes wider.

Expose

12. **Double-check everything.** Develop the habit of quickly reviewing major variables just before the exposure. Make sure that the retina is in focus. Double-check the flash setting. Monitor the IR screen image for even illumination and the absence of artifacts.
13. **Coach the patient.** Ask the patient to blink twice and then open his or her eyes very wide and keep them open.
14. **Expose the image.** Press down on the shutter release button to take a picture. (It's as easy as that!) The patient may sit back. Patients might complain that they cannot see out of that eye; reassure them that what they see is just like the spots they see when they look into a flash. Remind them that it is a big flash which covers the whole eye, so the spot is very large.
15. **Photograph the other eye.** You might need to wait 5–10 minutes to photograph the second eye because of the bright flash. Dilating drops minimize this time.
16. **Close the session.** Let your patients know that they did well (even if they did not) and that you obtained the needed photographs (which you should have). Remind them that the colors they are seeing are normal. Release the patient with a smile, making sure that he or she feels fine and knows where the next clinic stop is. Complete all paperwork, including signing the chart. To avoid confusion, finish completely with one patient before beginning another.

Follow-Up

17. **Label/archive your photographs.** Transfer or archive the images to the patient database if yours is a digital system (Fig. 2–10). Label each Polaroid with the patient's number, the date taken, and the requesting eye specialist. Some offices label each image with the patient's diagnosis.

18. **Deliver the finished product.** Insert prints or slides into the patient's chart or send files to the patient's electronic medical record (EMR) in a timely manner.

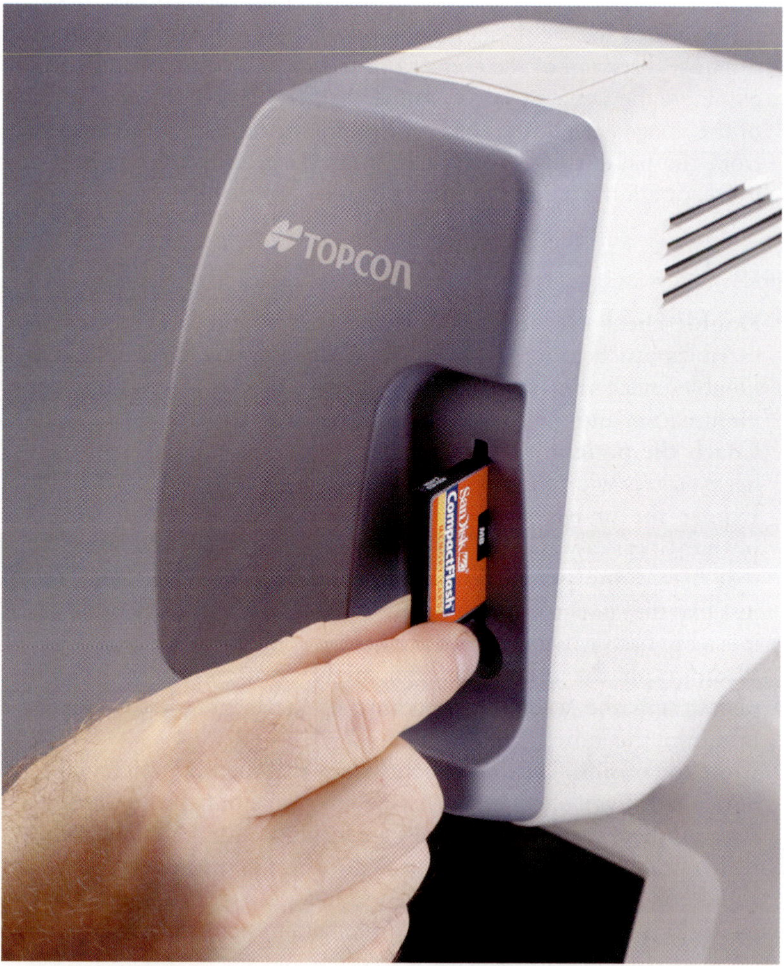

Figure 2–10 ○ Transfer the patient images from the nonmydriatic camera to your computer using a portable digital storage medium such as a compact flash or a micro-drive. Some nonmydriatic cameras feature a USB port for uploading images to your computer.

Chapter 3

Ten Fundus Photography FAQs*

Which Fundus Camera Should I Purchase?

It is a good idea to test-drive any major purchase. Review cameras at local practices, or take a workshop like those offered by the Ophthalmic Photographers' Society (www.opsweb.org). Here are some specific questions you should ask before purchasing any fundus camera.

- Is your practice general or specialized? Will this be your first or only fundus camera? If this is your second or third camera, consider either an identical fundus camera (for compatibility) (Fig. 3–1) or a decidedly different model (to expand photographic capabilities or take advantage of technological advances).
- Will the optics of this camera provide adequate or superior sharpness and contrast? Review actual clinical images, not just sales samples. What angles of view are available? How are the sharpness and contrast of each angle setting?
- What are your clinical needs? Will extremely fine macular detail be required in all images? Or is the camera to be used for general documentation?
- What type of patients will be photographed? Will their pupils be generally widely or poorly dilated? If your practice is primarily glaucoma, the patient population you will be photographing may have smaller pupils. What is the minimum pupil size required for a good fundus photograph on a particular camera model?
- Will patients be reasonably comfortable during the procedure? Sit in the patient's chair. Can physically challenged patients be accommodated? Is portability an issue? Will you need to move the camera between offices or to the operating room?

*Frequently asked questions.

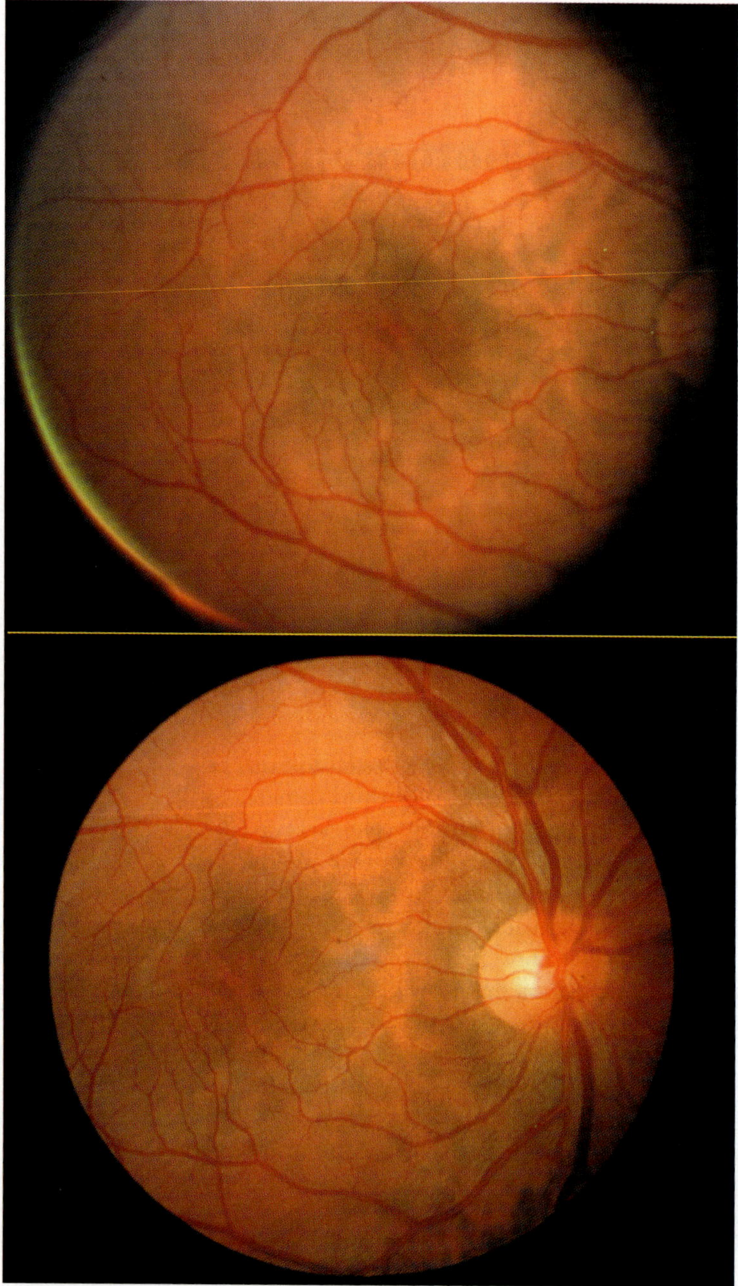

Figure 3–1 ○ Although these images are from cameras of identical optical design, it is probably not surprising that the image from the brand-new fundus camera (*bottom*) is sharper than the image from the older fundus camera (*top*), which has been moved, disassembled, and cleaned many times in 15 years.

- Are the camera's controls well balanced, adequately marked, and ergonomically well placed? How easy or difficult is the viewing or focusing system to use?
- Is this a reliable model? How sturdy does the camera feel? If this camera breaks down, how will it be repaired? What are the cost, expected life, and availability of viewing lamps and flash tubes?
- What is the initial cost of the unit? Is a used camera of the same model available?
- What experience have other photographers had with this camera model?
- Will the photographer using the camera be happy with it?

Which Film Should I Use?

Choosing a film involves multiple decisions. First, determine the general film type; then choose a specific brand (Fig. 3–2).

One way to describe film is by listing opposing characteristics. You already know that film is available in black-and-white and color varieties. It is also available as positive (slide film: black records as black) and negative film (black records as white). Of course, both black-and-white film and color film are available in positive and negative emulsions. Slow film (ISO 25: less sensitive to light but with a finer grain and better image quality) and fast film (ISO 400: more sensitive to light but with a coarser grain and lesser image quality) are options in each of the above categories. Finally, film can vary in its spectral sensitivity or light balance: Daylight, tungsten, and infrared emulsions are available. For routine fundus photography, most ophthalmic photographers choose a medium-speed (ISO 100) 35-mm color transparency film that is balanced for daylight.

Which specific brand or speed of film should you use? That question is best answered after individual testing. Although each film records physical reality, no pair of films ever records it in quite the same way. Each brand and speed of film has its own specific color cast and resolution (Fig. 3–3). The same brand of film (e.g., Kodachrome) is sold in different film speeds (e.g., 25, 64, and 200), each with slightly different image characteristics.

If you are unsure about the film characteristics described above, a basic photography course will help.

Film manufacturers are continually improving their film stocks. Keep current with emulsion changes, and test new films regularly.

Which Exposure Setting Should I Use?

Determining the correct exposure requires experimentation. First determine your standard exposure. Using a well-dilated volunteer and your standard film,

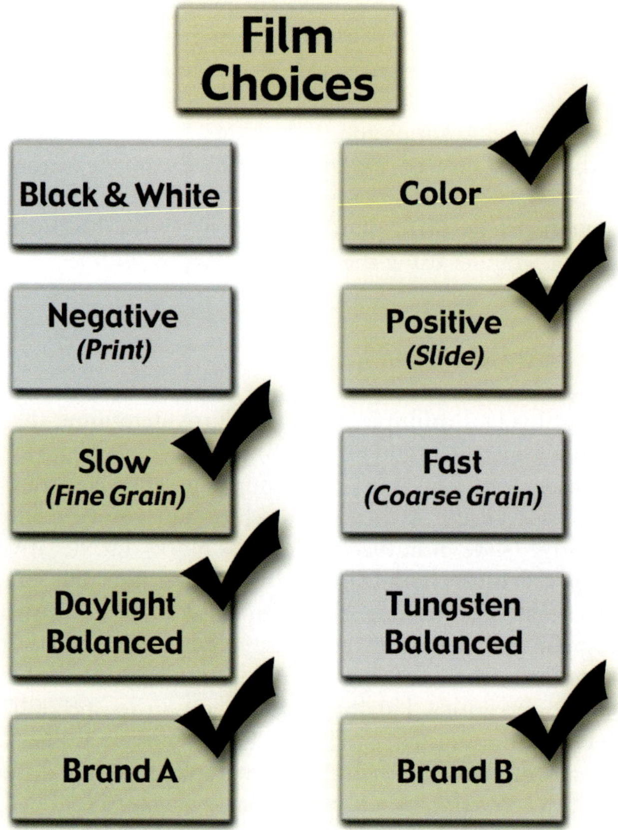

Figure 3–2 ○ With your final application in mind, follow the check marks: fundus photography requires a color film that is positive (slides), has a slow or medium speed (for fine grain), and is daylight-balanced (flash illumination). Once these broad characteristics have been defined, the choice of brand is a practical matter. Select the film with the best image quality, truest color balance, greatest convenience, and best value.

expose a fundus photograph at each of your flash settings (Fig. 3–4). Check the exposure at each angle of view. Review this series of photographs to determine the best standard exposure.

Use this standard exposure on all patients who have the same pupil and fundus coloration characteristics as your model. You might need to increase this exposure by one or two steps if a particular patient:

- Has a small pupil
- Has a retina with significantly darker pigmentation
- Has a large retinal hemorrhage

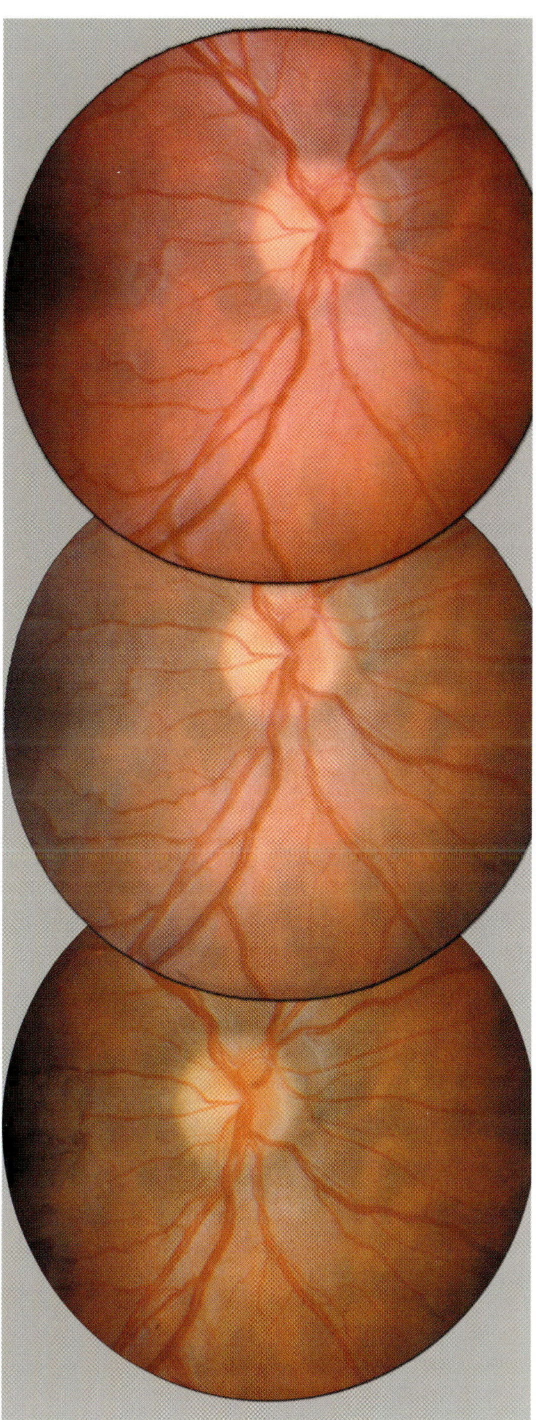

Figure 3–3 ○ Film and processing have a major impact on the color of your final fundus photographs. These three photographs of the same patient were exposed with the same camera on the same day but using different brands of film.

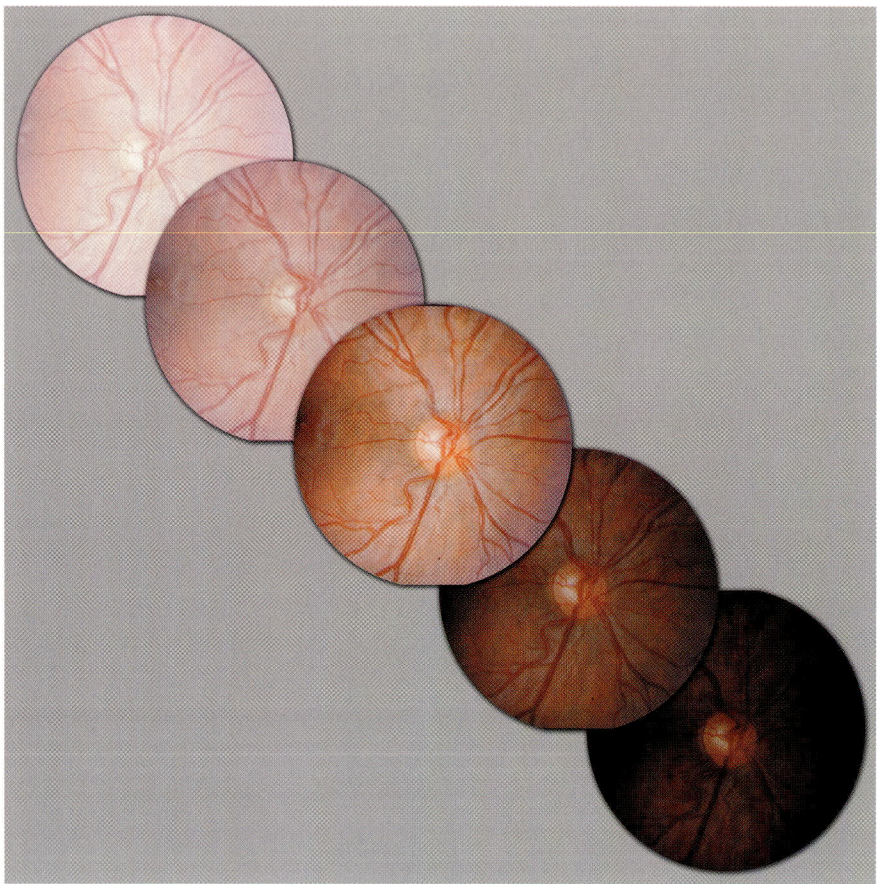

Figure 3–4 ○ Exposure test. Create a series of photographs using each of the flash settings on your power pack. Carefully evaluate the pictures to determine a standard exposure.

Decrease your exposure for:

- Young children
- Patients with significantly lighter pigmentation
- Patients with highly reflective fundi

Repeat this test each time you make a significant change in your procedure. Individually test each of your fundus cameras; each fundus camera–power supply combination will have unique exposure characteristics. If you notice an exposure drift toward darkened images over time, check the flash tube or schedule a thorough cleaning of your fundus camera.

How Should I Dilate My Patients?

High-quality fundus photography requires maximally dilated pupils (Fig. 3–5). The size of the pupil is controlled by the ciliary muscle, the iris sphincter muscle, and the dilating muscle. We manipulate the normal reactions of these muscles by using two different types of medications: mydriatics and cycloplegics (Table 3–1). Mydriatics are sympathomimetics that dilate the pupil (or affect mydriasis) by causing the dilator muscle to contract. They also cause vasoconstriction and should be used with caution in individuals with a history of hypertension or heart problems. A commonly used mydriatic is phenylephrine. Available in both 2.5% and 10% solutions, maximal pupil dilation begins in 20 minutes and lasts for approximately 3 hours.

Cycloplegics are parasympatholytics that cause mydriasis by relaxing the iris sphincter muscles. They also arrest accommodation (or cause cycloplegia) by paralyzing the ciliary muscle. A commonly used cycloplegic is tropicamide. Available in both 0.5% and 1% solutions, maximal pupil dilation occurs in approximately 30 minutes and lasts for 4–6 hours. Some offices prefer cyclopentolate. Available in 0.5%, 1%, and 2% solutions, it causes pupil dilation in 15-20 minutes and lasts for 24 hours. Other cycloplegics include atropine, homatropine, and scopolamine; each is available under various trade names.

Some important cautions: Read the medication insert completely for a description of contraindications and side effects. The administration of dilating drops is contraindicated in patients who are at risk for narrow-angle glaucoma. Estimate the anterior chamber depth before instilling dilation medication (Fig. 3–6). Check with your practitioner before dilating patients with iris-fixated intraocular lenses. Children and infants should be dilated by using ophthalmic medications that contain lower concentrations of active ingredients; consult with your practitioner for specific instructions.

Educate your patients about the normal side effects of dilation. Remind them that the drops might sting. Warn the patients of increased light sensitivity due to their enlarged pupils. Counsel your patients that reading may be difficult because their near vision will be blurry. Reassure them that their distance vision should not be affected. We always suggest that patients bring a driver if they will be dilated.

Begin by washing your hands with soap and water and instructing the patient to tilt his or her head back. Gently pull the lower eyelid down slightly to create a small space between the lid and the globe. Place a single drop in this pouch, being careful not to contaminate the bottle by allowing it to touch the patient. (The drop may be applied inside the lower eyelid, on the sclera, or on the cornea. The patient's blink will distribute the medication.) Instill a second drop if you are not sure that the first was successful. One properly placed drop is sufficient. After the drop has been instilled, ask the patient to close his or her

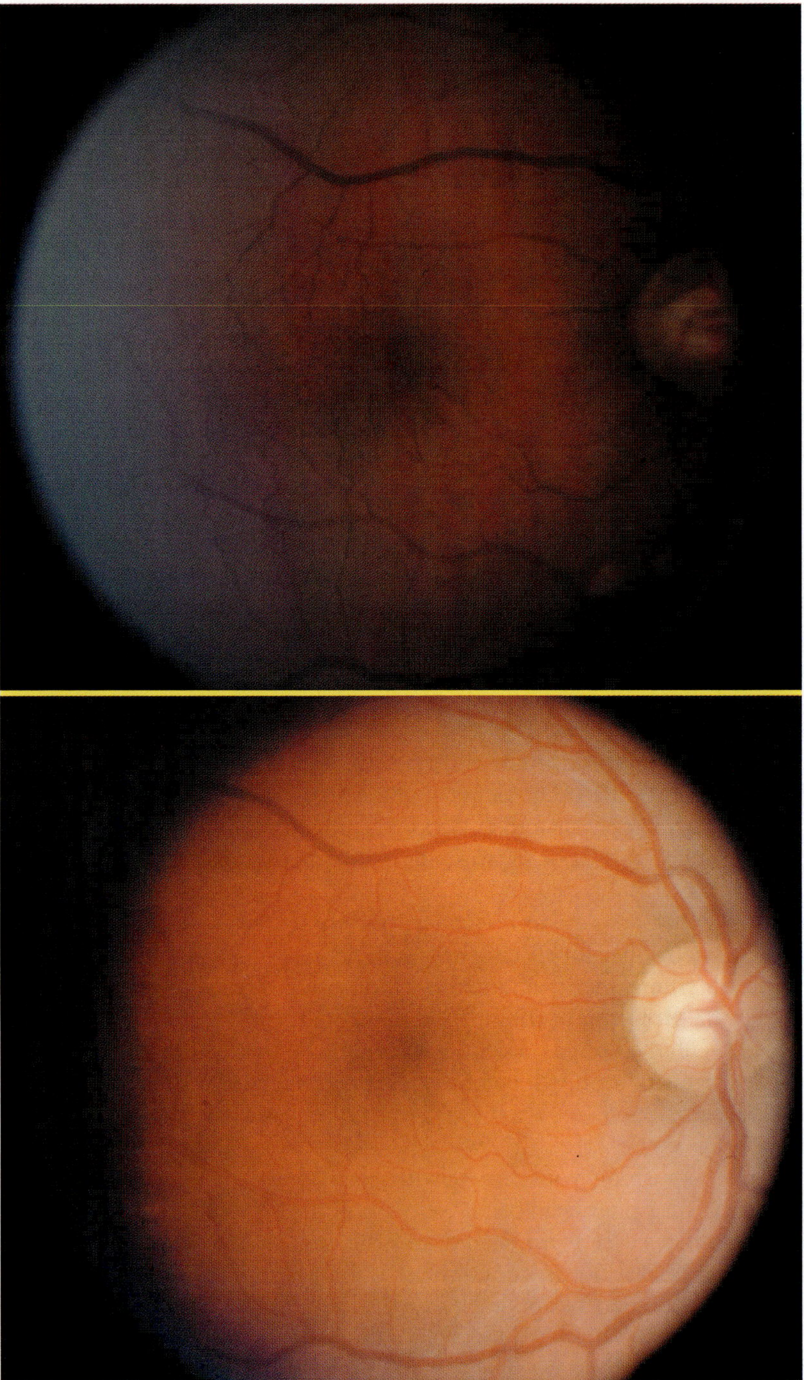

Figure 3–5 ○ Allow adequate time for your patient's eyes to dilate. Poor photographs (*top*) can be avoided if a full 20–30 minutes of dilation time (*bottom*) is allowed.

Table 3–1
Medications Used for Routine Dilation

Generic Name	Trade Name	Action	Maximal Effect	Duration
Tropicamide	Mydriacyl Opticyl Tropicacyl	Mydriasis and cycloplegia	20–30 min	4–6 hr
Cyclopentolate hydrochloride	AK-Pentolate Cyclogyl	Mydriasis and cycloplegia	15–30 min	24 hr
Phenylephrine hydrochloride	AK-Dilate Efricel Mydfrin Neo-Synephrine	Mydriasis	20–40 min	3 hr

eyes for a moment (without squeezing the eyelids). Patients may gently dab their closed eyes with a clean tissue but should avoid applying pressure. Wait a minute or two between different eye medications.

Pay careful attention to the expiration date of your dilating medications. Never instill outdated or discolored medication. Consider dating the bottles when opened and then disposing of opened bottles after 30 days.

Which Patient Chair Is Best?

Patient comfort and patient stability are two important considerations in selecting a patient chair. Height should be adjustable for multiple patient sizes, and seats should be wide and padded for large patients. Wheeled stools with backs allow mobility between multiple cameras in a single room; locking casters promote patient stability. Motorized reclining patient examination chairs (with footrests removed) have been adopted in many clinics.

Which Eye Should I Photograph First?

It matters little which eye you choose as long as you establish a logical and systematic approach to your patients. One convention suggests photographing the macula of the right eye (OD) first. This establishes a routine introduction to the patient both at the camera and at the editing table.

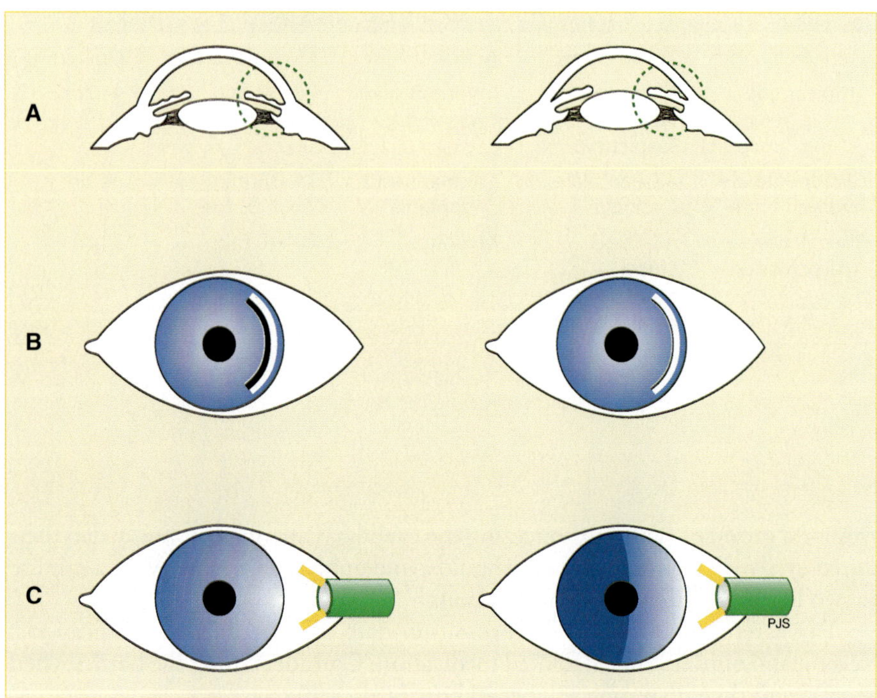

Figure 3–6 ○ Estimate the anterior chamber depth of each patient before introducing dilation medication. Normal anterior chambers will not close during routine dilation. Narrow anterior chamber angles, however, may close on routine dilation, causing increased intraocular pressure and the possibility of an episode of medication-induced closed-angle glaucoma. Anatomically, the normal iris is well separated from the trabecular network (*A*). The iris and trabecular meshwork are more closely positioned in patients with narrow angles. Angle depths are estimated by using a 0 (closed-angle) through 4 (large, fully open angle) scale. Slit-lamp examination is the best method for estimating anterior chamber depth. If a slit beam is projected at a 45-degree angle, then the aqueous space is indicated by unilluminated space (the black line between the two white lines) between the corneal reflection and the beam's projection on the iris (*B*). The normal anterior chamber will reveal a wide space; the narrow anterior chamber, a narrow distance. A flashlight projected at the limbus in the same plane as the iris can also be used to estimate the depth of the anterior chamber, although routine use of this technique has fallen out of favor with many professionals. Normal chambers cast little or no shadow. A bowed iris in a shallow anterior chamber projects a wide shadow across the pupil to the limbus (*C*). Careful slit-lamp or flashlight examination is necessary on all patients before dilation. Always check with an eye care professional before dilating a patient with a narrow anterior chamber angle.

Another approach is to photograph the affected eye first. The affected eye is the eye in which the practitioner is most interested. If the session ends early (e.g., if the camera breaks or if a very young patient declines further photography), then the most important images have been captured.

How Many Photographs Should I Take?

The answer to this question depends on the patient, your skill level, and your practice. Your goal is a sharp, well-exposed fundus photograph. Patients will routinely blink, shift fixation, move their heads, and in general make it difficult to guarantee that any single exposure will succeed. Most experienced photographers expose at least two photographs (or two stereo pairs) of each requested retinal field. It is less expensive to use an extra frame of film for insurance than to repeat the session. It may be difficult to expose multiple photographs of a young child or an extremely light-sensitive patient; attempt to capture the best single image you can.

Novice fundus photographers might need to expose more images to obtain a single good fundus photograph. This is encouraged: Experience is your best teacher.

Interesting or rare pathology deserves a few additional photographs. If you or someone in your practice routinely lectures or publishes, increase your number of exposures. Originals are always better than duplicate slides for teaching and publication.

On the other hand, digital imaging may reduce the need for multiple photographs. Once you have a fine image up on the screen, except for stereo imaging, there is really no reason to duplicate it.

You will need additional original exposures to build a portfolio of interesting patients. A portfolio is required for CRA (Certified Retinal Angiographer) certification and for most ophthalmic photography job interviews.

What If My Patient Can't Follow the External Fixation Light?

There are a number of reasons why your patient might not be able to fixate on the external fixation light. The most obvious one is that your patient probably has vision problems! Try one of the following practical suggestions:

- **Clarify your instructions.** Patients may look to the side and see the fixation light with the eye you are photographing. They will ask you which of the two lights you want them to look at—the one to the side or the one straight ahead. Ask them to look at the little light in the middle of the big light or at the small light straight ahead.

- **Change the visual stimulus.** Try moving the fixation light from side to side using short, quick movements. If your camera doesn't have a blinking fixation light, then simulate blinking by rapidly moving your finger back and forth in front of the fixation light.
- **Change the location of the fixation light.** Younger patients may cross their eyes. If your instructions to look straight ahead fail, try moving the fixation light closer to or farther away from the patient. Some patients will straighten their eyes if you move the fixation light farther away, effectively hiding it from the eye being photographed. Alternatively, move the fixation light closer to the inner canthus. The fixating eye will remain crossed, but the eye being photographed will be looking straight ahead.
- **Use the internal fixation device.** This stick will look in focus to the patient when it looks in focus to you (Fig. 3–7). Remove the internal fixation device before the fundus photograph is exposed.
- **Instruct the patient verbally.** If you have difficulty obtaining fixation with either fixation target, try asking the patient to look straight ahead in the middle of the light for macula views. Simple directions (left, right, up, and down) or clock hours will help with peripheral views.

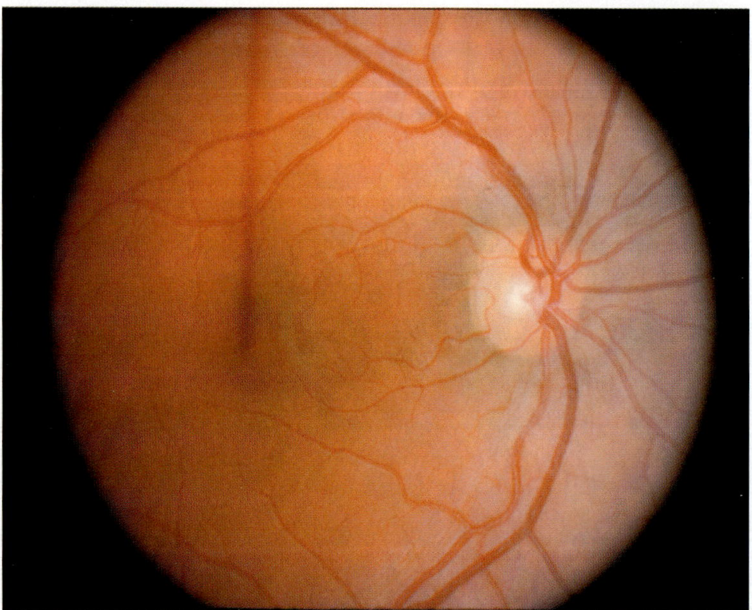

Figure 3–7 ○ The internal fixation target documents the point of fixation but also obscures macular detail, so in most cases it should be removed just prior to exposing the photograph.

- **Move the camera.** If you cannot obtain reliable fixation, simply instruct the patient to hold his or her eyes still. Use your fundus camera's adjustments to swing, tilt, or otherwise move until you locate the area of interest.
- **Do your best.** Some of your most challenging patients will be those who could not be examined. Use your widest angle of view for young patients who may not have reliable fixation. Define a null point (the position of gaze at which the patient's eye movement decreases or stops) in patients with nystagmus, or time your photographs to coincide with the patient's eye movements just before the eye changes direction.

My Pictures Are Blurry. What Should I Do?

Blurry fundus photographs of patients without media problems are often the result of the photographer accommodating during the procedure (Fig. 3–8). Accommodation is the normal mechanism your eye uses for focusing on near objects. In simple terms, the ciliary muscle tugs or releases tension on the lens zonules, modifying the refractive power of the lens. At the same time, the near reflex causes miosis and convergence. The ability to accommodate lessens with age.

When you look through the camera eyepiece and accommodate, you might see a sharp image of the retina but not see a sharp image of the focusing reticle. If you accommodate to obtain a sharp retinal image, then the optical system of your eye, rather than the optical system of the fundus camera, is used to obtain sharpness. You might attempt to sharpen the image using the focusing knob, but the result will be a blurry photograph.

The tendency to accommodate when focusing occurs in fatigued and novice fundus photographers and in experienced photographers who are younger than approximately 40 years of age. Strategies for safeguarding against accommodation problems during procedures include the following:

- You can feel yourself accommodate. Find a quiet room with no distractions. Fully relax your mind and body while focusing your eyes on an object at least 20 feet away. Bring your index finger approximately 18 inches from your nose. When you focus on your index finger, notice that the background becomes unsharp. Keeping your finger in focus, move it toward your nose slowly. The background will become increasingly less sharp, and the edges of your visual field will constrict. You will feel your eyes converge, and you might feel a sensation in the anterior section of your eyes. Focus on the distant object again and repeat. With practice, you will become more aware of your personal sensation during accommodation. If you feel this sensation during fundus photography, an unsharp photograph may result.

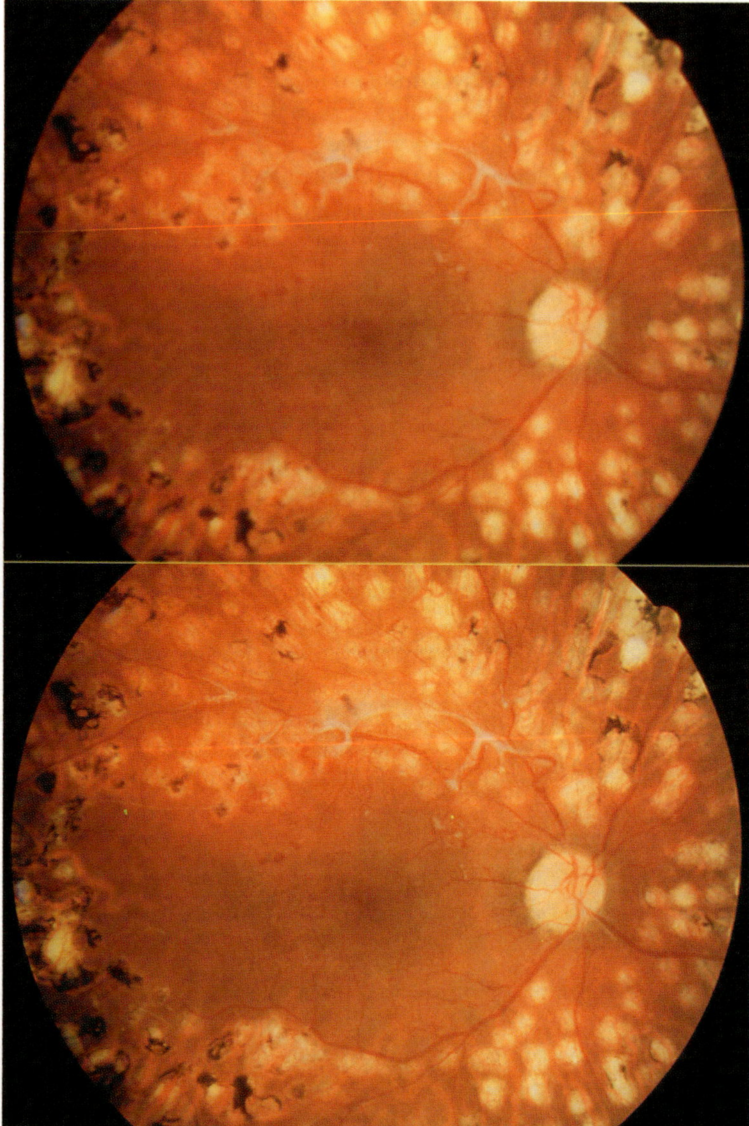

Figure 3–8 ○ A blurry image (*top*) results from an otherwise clear patient (*bottom*) when the fundus photographer has not carefully set the eyepiece reticle and carefully used the reticle while focusing.

- If you think you are accommodating during a procedure, look away from the eyepiece. Blink or close your eyes to help reset their focus. On looking again into the viewfinder, concentrate on the thin black lines of the focusing reticle.
- Try to keep both eyes open throughout the procedure, preferably with the non-eyepiece eye focused across the room.
- A full day of fundus photography may distort the normal accommodative process, causing your eye to be "stuck" in near focus. Accommodative excess is the result of prolonged and intense periods of near work, which may result in eyestrain and headaches.

Of course, your eyes should always be corrected to their best visual acuity. You might find that one eye is sharper than the other. Keep your eyeglasses or contact lenses scrupulously clean. Dry eyes can be a problem if you find yourself blinking less frequently when looking through the viewfinder. Use artificial tears or contact lens wetting solution as needed.

To fully understand the fine points of focusing, review Chapter 5, "Focusing the Fundus Camera."

How Should I Clean My Fundus Camera?

The best fundus photographs are taken by using a fundus camera with a clean front element (Fig. 3–9). Obtain specific cleaning recommendations from your fundus camera manufacturer. Most lenses will not be harmed by over-the-counter "photographic" or "coated lens" cleaners and good-quality photographic lens cleaning tissue. Avoid products that leave an obvious residue.

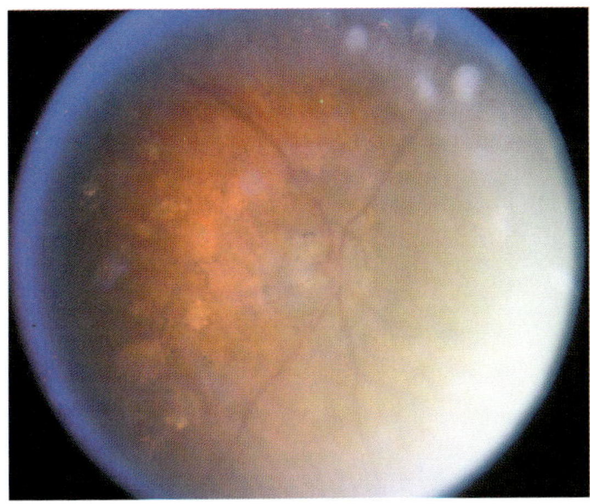

Figure 3–9 ○ This fundus photograph was not taken during a blizzard. Keep your front element scrupulously clean. Blurry white circles appearing in the image are images of dust, dirt, or tears on the front of your objective lens.

Begin by inserting the negative diopter lens and focusing on the dust on the front element. Use a bulb syringe to blow off any loose dust. Place a few drops of lens-cleaning solution on a piece of lens tissue or natural cotton (never on the lens itself and never on a commercial cotton swab manufactured with glue). Using gentle pressure, wipe in circular motions, beginning in the center of the lens and spiraling to the outside. Follow each damp lens tissue with a dry one, wiping in the same motion. It may take a few passes to clean your lens well; be patient and resist the urge to scrub the glass. Complete the process by breathing gently on the lens before the final wipe with a dry lens cleaning tissue.

Use common sense when cleaning your camera's lens. Clean regularly (but not after each patient) and gently (not vigorously).

After cleaning, the best way to keep your front element clean is to actively use the lens cap. Place the lens cap over the lens between each patient and whenever you leave the room—even when changing film!

Have your optics checked regularly by the manufacturer's service technician. Refer the cleaning of internal optics to a trained professional.

Of course, your front element is not the only place your fundus camera needs to be cleaned. External surfaces that come into contact with your patients should be disinfected both after each patient and at the end of the day.

What's Wrong with My Pictures?

The ideal fundus photograph is an accurate visual representation of the retina. Of course, as with any complex process, many things may go wrong (Fig. 3–10). Artifacts are portions of the image that arise from the process, not from the patient's retina. Typical artifacts include yellow or orange crescents, white or blue haze at the edge of the photograph, blinks, dust on the front element, and poor focus.

If artifacts are described systematically, we learn about the subtleties of the image and will more likely reason or intuit the artifact's cause. The first step in determining the cause of fundus photograph errors is accurately describing the artifact. Four essential details help to describe the artifact: the extent, character, distribution, and frequency of the affected slide (Table 3–2, Fig. 3–11).

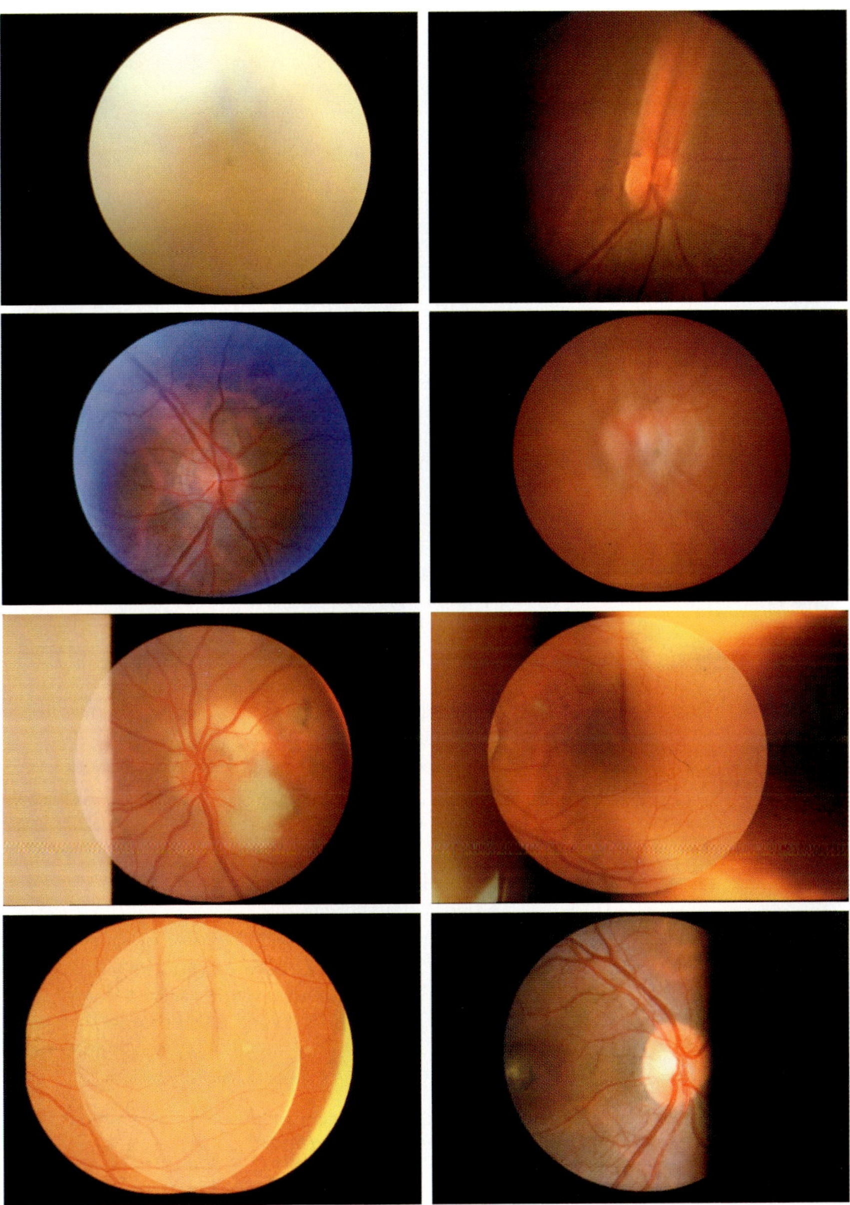

Figure 3–10 ○ Artifacts can arise from each part of the process. The patient may blink (*top left*) or have too many tears (*top right*). The patient may have a small pupil, which causes a blue-tinted glare from their IOL (*second left*), or a small IOL and large pupil, which cause a double image (*second right*). The photographer may forget to take two or three exposures when loading the film (*third left*) or may inadvertently open the camera back without rewinding the film (*third right*). The camera motor may malfunction, causing a double exposure (*bottom left*), or the shutter speed can be on the wrong setting, causing the shutter curtain to hide part of the image (*bottom right*).

Table 3–2
Descriptors for Fundus Photography Artifacts

Extent	Full frame	There is no useful information in any part of the frame. The picture may be completely black or white.
	Full image area	The standard fundus image area contains no useful information, but the black surround (unexposed because of the fundus camera's mask) and the film frame numbers are left unaffected.
	Partial image area	The artifact obscures a portion of the retinal image area; the remaining retinal image is of adequate quality.
Character	Location	The artifact can be described as central or peripheral; superior, inferior; to the right or left.
	Shape	Circular, crescent-shaped, or rectangular artifacts with sharp or blurry borders are possible.
	Exposure	The overall photograph may be too light or dark, or it may be a double exposure.
	Color	The artifact may be any color; white, yellow, orange, and blue are common. Multicolored artifacts are also seen.
	Sharpness	The full image area may be sharp or unsharp, as can portions thereof.
Distribution		The artifact can be found at the beginning, the middle, or the end of the roll.
Frequency		The artifact may be observed randomly or regularly, throughout a single roll or a single patient, or crossing several rolls or patients. Artifacts can be seen frequently, occasionally, or just once.

Note: Providing a complete description of fundus photography artifacts helps us reason or intuit their cause. Use the vocabulary from this table when describing artifacts.

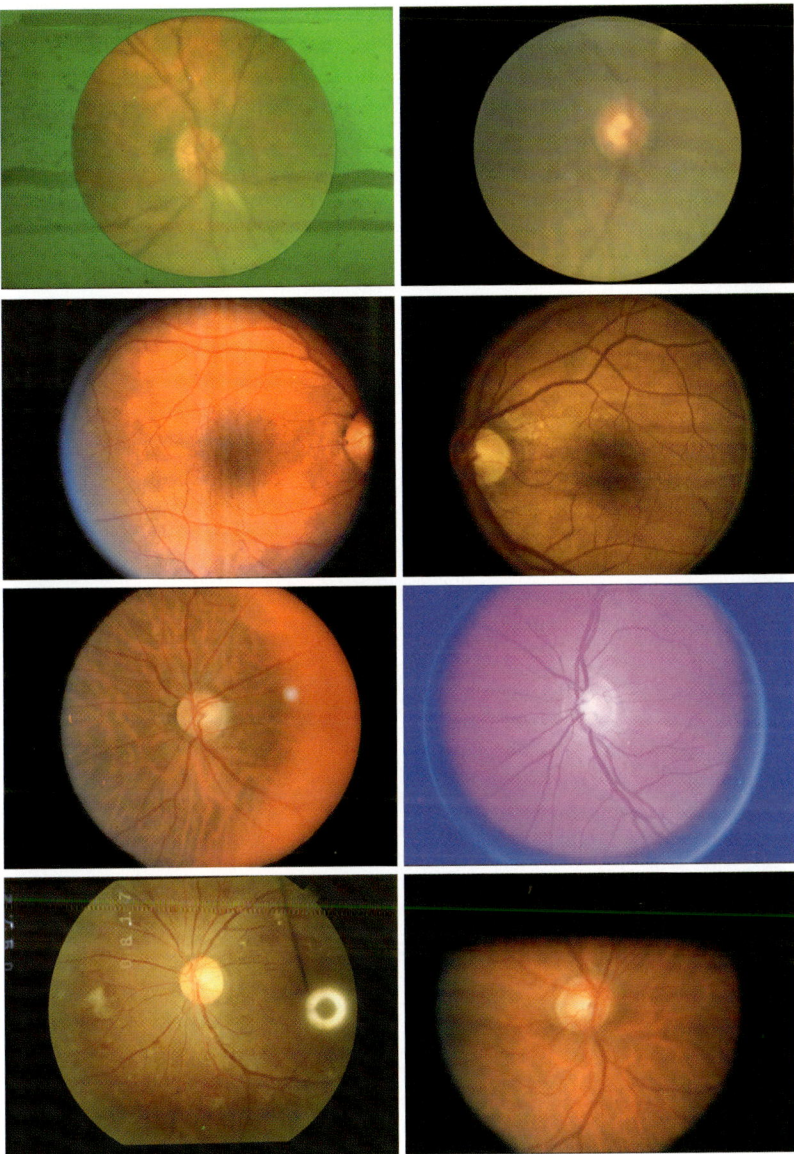

Figure 3–11 ○ Examples of a standard vocabulary for describing fundus photography artifacts. Extent: The full frame of this fundus photograph is discolored from a processing error (*top left*), while only the image area is discolored in this patient with a vitreous hemorrhage (*top right*). Character: The vertical stripes are the result of rewinding the film backward (second left), while the horizontal stripes are chemical streaks (*second right*). Frequency: A crescent-shaped artifact will occur without regularity, but a dust spot (the small white circular artifact) will occur in every frame until the lens is cleaned (*third left*). Every patient's fundus photograph will be discolored if it is exposed with out-of-date film, which fades (*third right*). Distribution: The bright circular reflection of a misaligned angle-changing lever (bottom left) may occur only when a certain angle of view is selected. The shadow from a slow single-lens reflex mirror (*bottom right*) will show in every patient's photograph until the problem is corrected.

Chapter 4

The Challenging Fundus Photograph

With practice, successful fundus photography of a cooperative patient with clear media and widely dilated pupils becomes routine. Not all patients are ideal, however. Patients with glaucoma and diabetes generally have smaller pupils. Elderly patients often have cataracts. And light-sensitive patients may have difficulty cooperating. In many clinics, fundus photography is performed at the end of the patient's appointment. By the time patients are ready to be photographed, they are tired and irritable. What is the best way to take successful photographs in these difficult clinical situations? This chapter suggests some solutions to common challenges.

Illumination Problems

Maximum pupil dilation allows the entrance and exit of illuminating and imaging light rays without mutual interference. Establish a dilating regimen that is safe and provides adequate dilation for fundus photography. Expect widely dilated pupils in young patients who are not taking medications, especially if they have light irises. Expect smaller pupils in older patients, in patients who have diabetes or who are being medicated for glaucoma, and in patients with dark irises. Less than maximum dilation will impair accurate focusing and alignment.

Your images may be locally underexposed, especially with wide-angle fundus cameras (Fig. 4–1). Increase your flash setting, choose a smaller angle of view, or insert the small-pupil diaphragm for a more evenly illuminated final photograph. Decentering the fundus camera may result in better illumination (Fig. 4–2). As a last resort, if the black cloud continues to persist, avoid placing it over important pathology.

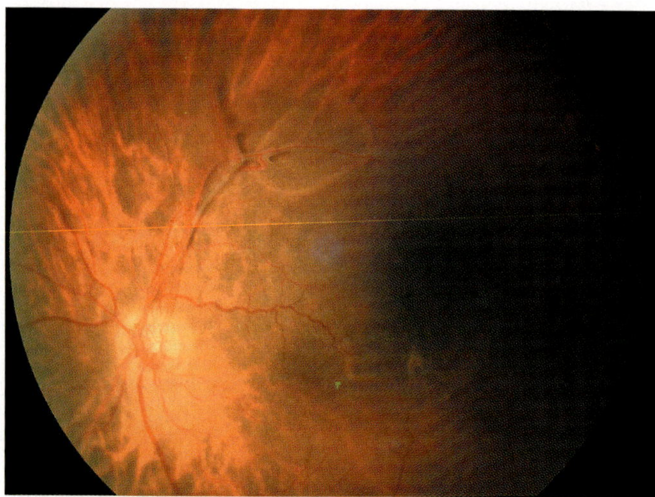

Figure 4–1 ○ Dark clouds. If a patient's pupil is significantly smaller than the outer diameter of the illuminating doughnut, a portion of the retina will receive inadequate illumination. The resultant "dark cloud" shifts as the camera's position changes. If you cannot eliminate the underexposed area, minimize its interaction with pathology.

Unsharp Subjects

The bundle of illuminating and imaging rays must pass twice through the patient's tear film, cornea, anterior chamber, lens, and vitreous. The clarity of the final fundus photograph is directly related to the clarity of each of these layers.

Specific areas of the cornea and lens may affect the passage of light. Maneuver around local areas of unsharpness such as central cataracts, corneal scars, and pterygia. The key to success is positioning the central imaging light rays through a clear portion of the media (Fig. 4–3). Spend time exploring all possible camera positions.

A dry, swollen, or hazy cornea, asteroid hyalosis, and vitreous hemorrhage represent conditions that can blur the entire fundus photograph. Adequate tear film is essential for corneal clarity and a sharp fundus image (Fig. 4–4). Encourage your patients to blink frequently. Instill artificial tears in patients with dry corneas. Applying glycerin topically (under the physician's supervision and with a topical anesthetic) to an edematous cornea may help sharpen the image.[1]

Corneal manipulation diminishes corneal clarity. Applanation tonometry disturbs the corneal epithelium and discolors the cornea with topical fluorescein. Examination with diagnostic contact lenses may cause slight corneal edema and introduce topical methylcellulose. Fundus photography should be performed before any procedure that involves corneal applanation. If postlaser photographs

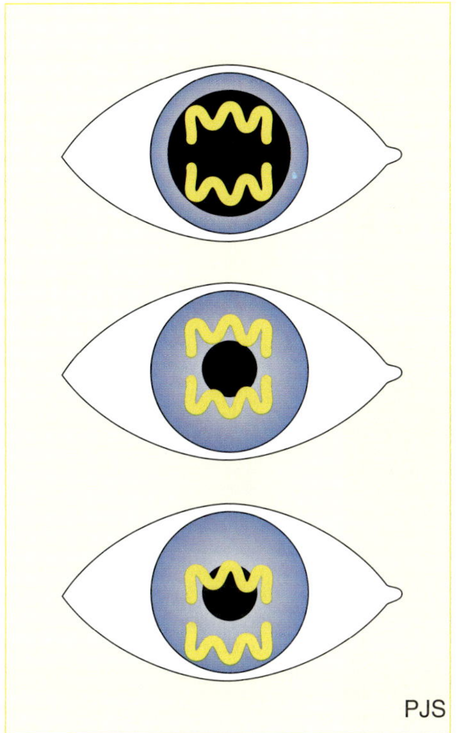

PJS

Figure 4–2 ○ Decentering the fundus camera may help to illuminate the fundus through a small pupil. Normally, the doughnut of the viewing light fits readily within the dilated pupil when centered (*top*). If the dilated pupil is very small, centering the doughnut may exclude illumination (*center*). Lowering or raising the camera axis (*bottom*) again divides the pupil evenly between viewing illumination and imaging rays. Be sure to increase the exposure to compensate for the smaller amount of illumination.

are requested, rinse the cornea multiple times with a commercially available eyewash preparation.

There is little you can do to sharpen the final photograph if dense asteroid hyalosis, vitreous hemorrhage, or a mature cataract exists. Indeed, obtaining a view of the retina can be a feat in itself. When general haziness is a problem, focus with a green filter (540–570 nm) to help increase the contrast between the blood vessels and the retina. If you cannot distinguish blood vessels, begin by locating the disc; it will look like a bright, blurry circle. Focus as best you can, and then, using the disc as your landmark, locate the requested field. Your final photograph will almost always contain retinal details that are not perceived through the viewfinder (Fig. 4–5).

Document hazy media or a small pupil with an external photograph. Adjust the fundus camera by moving the patient's headrest away from the objective lens, inserting the plus diopter setting, and increasing the exposure. Focus on the level of the opacity. Use the optic disc as a reflector by centering it directly behind the pupil.

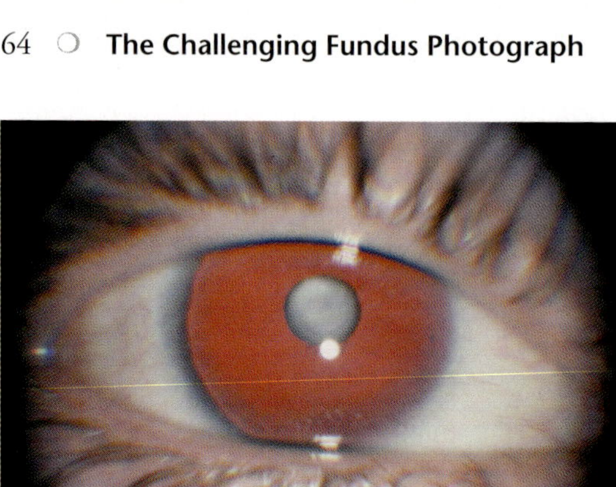

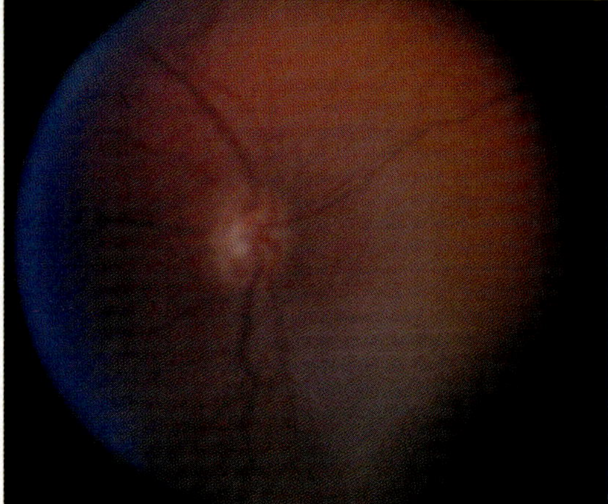

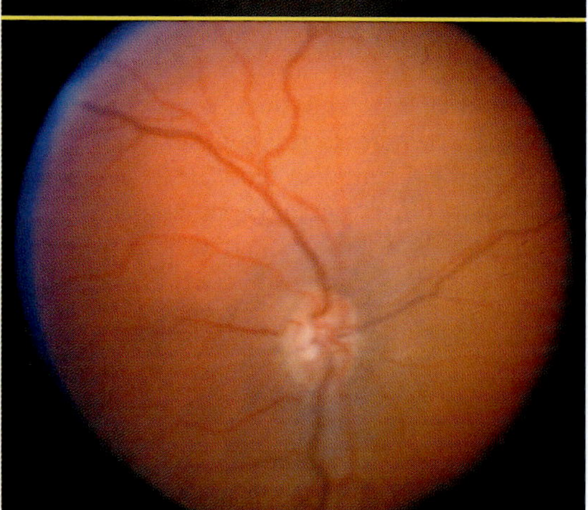

Figure 4–3 ○ Look for local areas of sharpness in patients with cataracts (*top*). Initial central alignment gave a blurry fundus photograph (*center*), but careful searching revealed a clearer view (*bottom*).

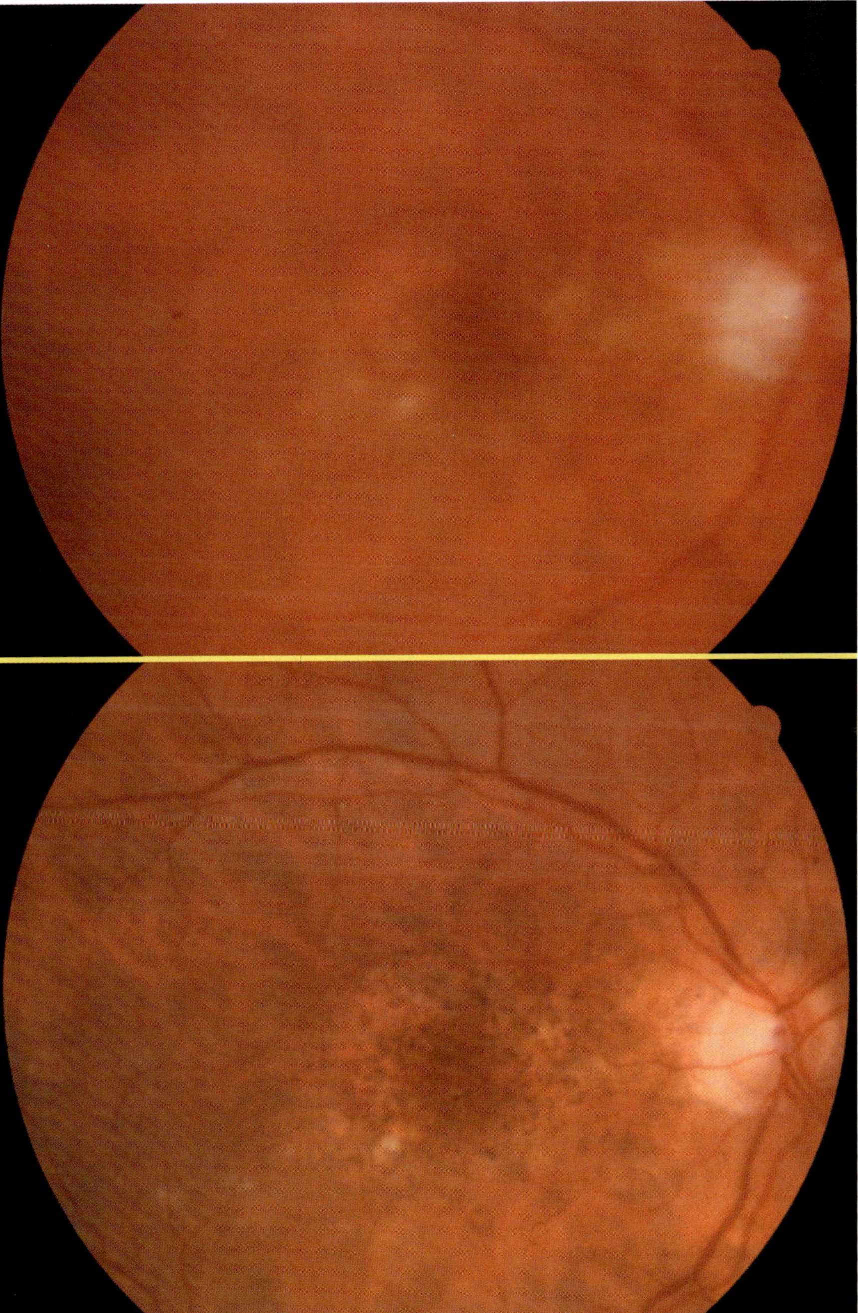

Figure 4–4 ○ Adequate tear film is essential for a clear fundus photograph. A blurry view (*top*) can be transformed into a much clearer photograph (*bottom*) by asking the patient to blink twice.

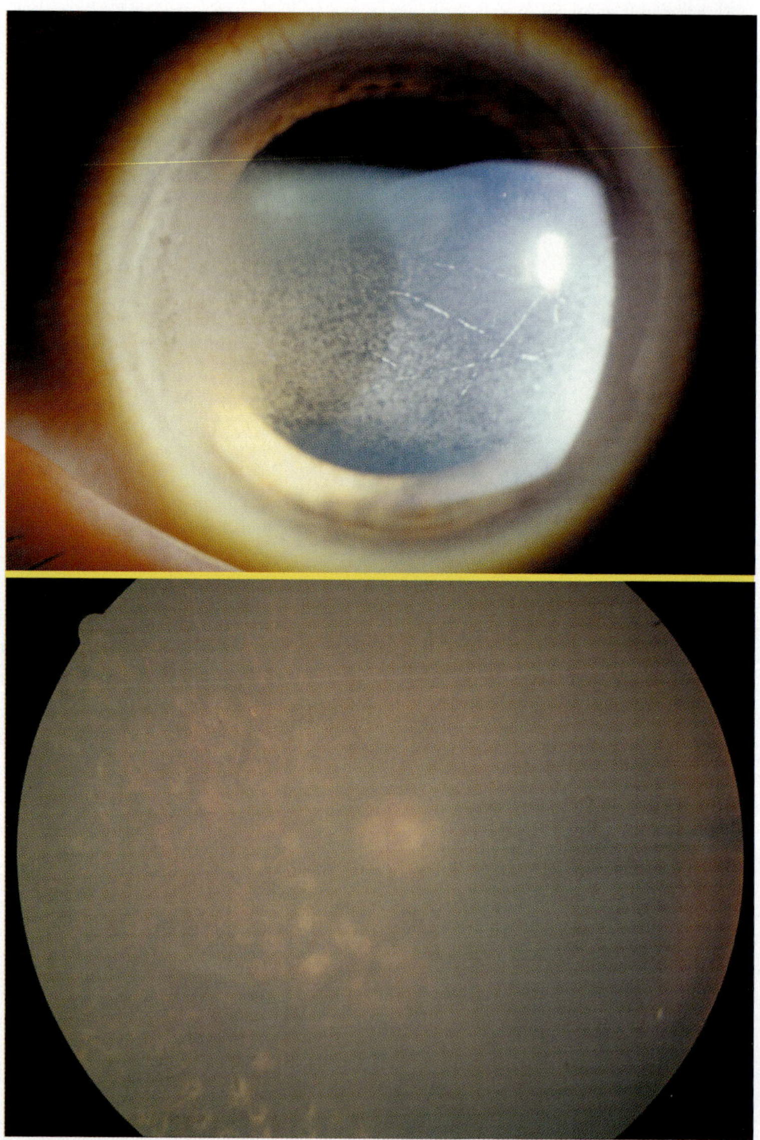

Figure 4–5 ○ The fundus photography in an eye with compromised media (*top*) might not be a prize winner, but it may contain adequate diagnostic information (*bottom*).

The Light-Sensitive Patient

Most people have a natural aversion to bright lights. Light-sensitive patients blink and tear excessively when looking into the fundus camera. Younger patients are often more light sensitive than older patients. Aphakic and pseudophakic patients are in general more light sensitive, having lost the filtering qualities of their natural lens. Patients with cataracts may be quite light sensitive. Patients with cone dystrophy, albinism, or blepharospasm may be extremely light sensitive. Avoidance behavior by these patients may make camera alignment difficult.

Prepare your patient for multiple bright flashes by accurately explaining the procedure. Inform the light-sensitive patient of your progress throughout the photographic session, and provide copious amounts of verbal encouragement and praise. Patients may complain of dry corneas; instill artificial tears in both eyes to reduce discomfort of dry corneas. An alternative option for the frequent blinker and light-sensitive patient is a drop of topical anesthetic.

Many fundus cameras have an illumination intensity knob that adjusts the focusing illumination from virtually nil to very bright. Use the lowest illuminating intensity at which you can clearly distinguish retinal detail. You might find it useful to turn the viewing light up while focusing and then down to a minimal level while photographing.

The light-sensitive patient might more easily tolerate focusing when a green filter (540–570 nm) is placed in the illumination path. Remove the filter just before the exposure.

Be constantly aware of your patient's disposition throughout the procedure. Frequent rest breaks (between, not within, stereo pairs) help keep the patient fresh. Tension-relieving techniques, including deep breathing, shoulder relaxation, and humor, are useful. Remember that patients are usually trying to do their best—even when it seems that they are not. Use positive reinforcement and praise to help your patients work with you rather than against you.

Patients will often adjust their disposition according to your behavioral cues. If you exhibit calmness and patience, your patient will make an effort in that direction. If you become exasperated and exhibit obnoxious behavior, your patient will often react in a like manner. Don't be afraid to call a time-out if either you or the patient needs some time to regain composure.

Eyelids

A cooperative light-sensitive patient will allow you to lift his or her upper eyelid with a cotton-tipped applicator. An uncooperative light-sensitive patient will require you to depend on an assistant to hold both the upper and lower lids. Use cotton-tipped applicators or a gloved finger for lid manipulation. Place the tip of an applicator at the bottom of the upper lid and rotate it up and in to raise the lid (Fig. 4–6). Rotate the swab clockwise (as seen temporally) for the right eye and counterclockwise for the left eye. Do not depress the globe during lid manipulation, as this may induce astigmatism.

Lid speculum use is not usually recommended; it may cause corneal abrasion in an uncooperative patient. Some photographers suggest that the patient hold his or her own eyelids.[2] Be aware that the patient may be more interested in avoiding bright lights than in ensuring that the procedure is successfully completed.

Eyelids may present a mechanical (rather than behavioral) barrier to fundus photography. Lid elevation is necessary for the patient with blepharoptosis. Manage excess eyelid skin with the creative use of tape (Fig. 4–7).

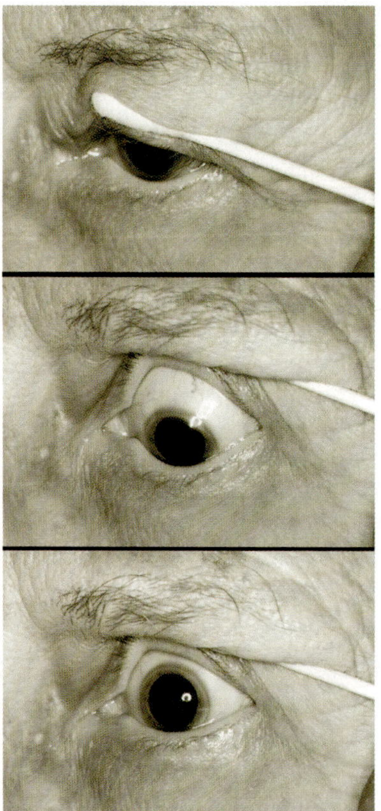

Figure 4–6 ○ To retract the upper lids with a cotton-tipped applicator, have the patient look down, and place the cotton tip at the lid margin (*top*). Rotate the applicator (clockwise right eye, counterclockwise left eye) (*middle*). Instruct the patient to look straight ahead (*bottom*), and continue fundus photography.

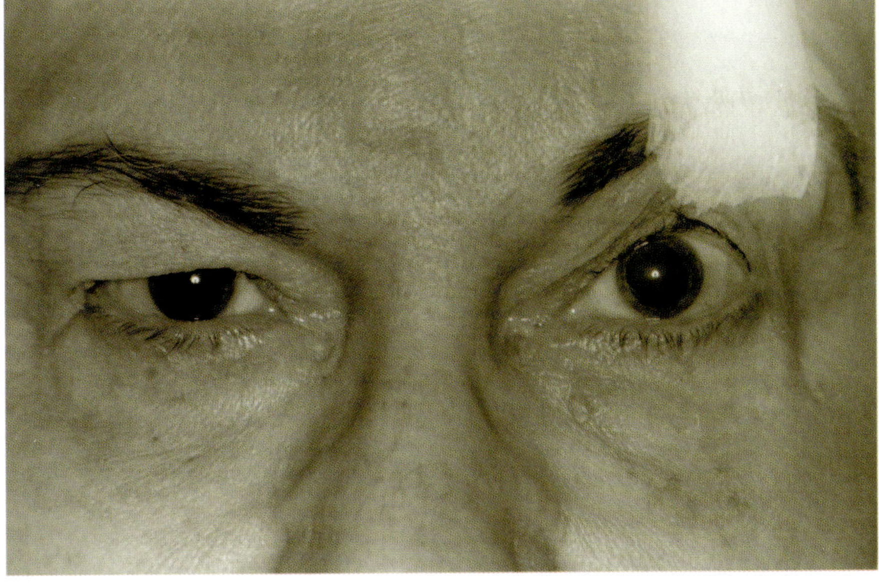

Figure 4–7 ○ "Instant lid lifts" with adhesive tape are useful with some ptotic eyelids.

Children

Retinal photography challenges quickly mount when the patient is a child. One difficulty is that the equipment is designed for the "average-sized" adult. Successful patient management techniques for the young patient vary with the age of the patient. Infants, toddlers, grade-schoolers, and teenagers all require specific strategies.

Babies are both the easiest and most difficult patients to photograph. Those who have just been fed are cooperative and sleepy, while those who are hungry or have missed their naps are invariably cranky and challenging. Patience and good humor are your only means of taming the uncooperative child. Your most emotionally challenging photographic subjects will be the retinas of children who have been abused.

For babies, use a hand-held fundus camera. Alternatively, the forehead rest may be removed from the standard-angle fundus camera and your young patients laid on their side.[3] A pediatric speculum provides access to the pupil. Speculum use requires topical anesthesia and a balanced salt solution to keep the cornea moist. A standard mummy wrap with two or three volunteers (for head, torso, and legs) stabilizes the child. Remember to take into account both the decreased pupil size and the shorter axial length in children younger than 3 years old when setting your flash exposure. Expose several photographs if you can, bracketing toward the lower flash settings. Use your general or external camera and flash to document abnormalities in abused children.

Use verbal communication to your advantage with toddlers and grade-schoolers. Speak directly to the patient, rather than communicating through the parent. Introduce yourself directly to the child with a smile to help establish trust. Remind young children of the special events (such as birthdays or holidays) that are usually associated with picture taking. Explain the intended procedure as being just as necessary (using a nod and eye contact to make sure the parents understand). Speak slowly and distinctly. Although all patients like to know what to expect, young children especially fear the unknown. Sharing a frank overview of the process informs children and allays their fears. Let your patient have some fun; our young patients like to experience photography from the "taking" end. We waste a frame of film but gain their friendship by letting them press the shutter release. An instant film image or digital print may be used to elicit a cooperative spirit and creates a great giveaway for show-and-tell. Spend as much time as needed to obtain the best photographs.

Difficulties may be encountered during your straightforward attempts at photography. Remember to respect each family's specific disciplinary system. Don't bribe or threaten to punish; other alternatives are available. Games help to focus the child's attention on something other than the procedure. The child might "pretend to be a statue" or "find the bunny in the middle of the lens."

Try setting a mutual goal with the patient. Ask the child to count aloud with you to three. Tell the child you will be taking three pictures and have him or her count each one along with you. You might want to cushion this figure; most children will allow only the negotiated number.

Actively solicit suggestions from the patient. Ask the child, "What can I do to make this easier for you?" Appeal to the child's friendship with the doctor or parent ("Dr. ____ thinks these pictures are important. Will you help me get them?"). If eyelids need to be held, employ a technician who has previously worked well with the particular child. Above all, remain calm and patient throughout the procedure.

Older children who are difficult may require you to announce, in a firm voice, "We need to take these pictures before you leave. Let's work together to get this completed." If you feel yourself losing control of the situation, sometimes it is better to leave the room and have the parent and child negotiate the terms of pictures. Be sure to leave with these verbal messages: "Dr. ____ thinks these pictures are important. When I come back, we'll be ready to finish the pictures." On returning to one 6-year-old girl, I discovered that the parent had agreed to pay the child $1.00 for each of three photographs.

It is especially important not to distress the child if you see the patient before the practitioner has completed the examination. As important as good photographs are, the doctor's examination takes precedence. However, the photographer may be the last health professional to see the child on a particular day. You have the opportunity to make future visits easier by parting with the patient on good terms.

Patient Communication

During fundus photography, the patient and photographer are thrust together for a brief time during which the photographer explores a very private part of the patient: the eyes. In this setting, the photographer must act in a variety of technical and communicative roles. Besides obtaining technically correct photographs, the photographer acts as the initiator, information giver, and coordinator. Ophthalmic photographers must be good communicators.

Show your patients respect by calling them from the waiting room using their first and last name and addressing them with their title (Mr./Mrs./Ms.) as appropriate. Be aware of the patient's body language throughout the procedure. Make conscious use of your body language, voice, word choice, and touch to keep your patients and their companions at ease. Be generous with positive feedback, especially if the patient is having trouble with the procedure. Keep a smile in your voice.

Communicate with patients using plain, straightforward English. Avoid street lingo and medical jargon. If the patient does not speak English, arrange for a translator. A relative or friend might be available, or your medical center or clinic might keep a list of employees with second-language talents. Keep in mind that a certified medical translator may be required for some procedures.

References

1. Wong D: Textbook of Ophthalmic Photography. New York: Inter-Optics Publications, 1982, p. 67.
2. Coppinger JM, Maio M, Miller K: Ophthalmic Photography. Thorofare, NJ: Slack, 1987, p. 89.
3. Szirth BC, Murphee AL, McNamara W: Infant fundus photography. J Ophthalmol Photog 1985;8:30.

Chapter 5

Focusing the Fundus Camera

Fundus photography is a system of information transfer: Visual information describing the clinical condition of the retina is transferred onto film. This visual representation is used by the practitioner to judge the health of the patient's retina and evaluate its treatment. Your goal is an accurate representation of the three-dimensional retinal and choroidal tissues. A sharp, well-focused retinal image is essential to successful fundus photography.

This chapter will show you how to obtain sharp fundus photographs and will describe the fundus camera's aerial image-focusing system. Proper focusing technique is related to retinal anatomy and pathology.

The Fundus Camera's Focusing System

In their most basic form, optical systems require light, a subject, a lens, a receiving plane, and an observer. Light reflects off the subject, is refracted by the lens, and is projected onto a receiving plane, where it is viewed. During fundus photography, the patient's retina becomes the subject, the optics of the patient's eye and the fundus camera replace the simple lens, the focusing screen or the film becomes the receiving plane, and you, the photographer, become the observer (Fig. 5–1). Focusing the fundus camera consists of adjusting the relationship between the subject and lens so that the subject lies within the depth of field of the lens and the receiving plane lies within the depth of focus of the image.

Most fundus cameras use a single-lens reflex (SLR) viewing system. Familiarize yourself with the basic SLR design (Fig. 5–2).

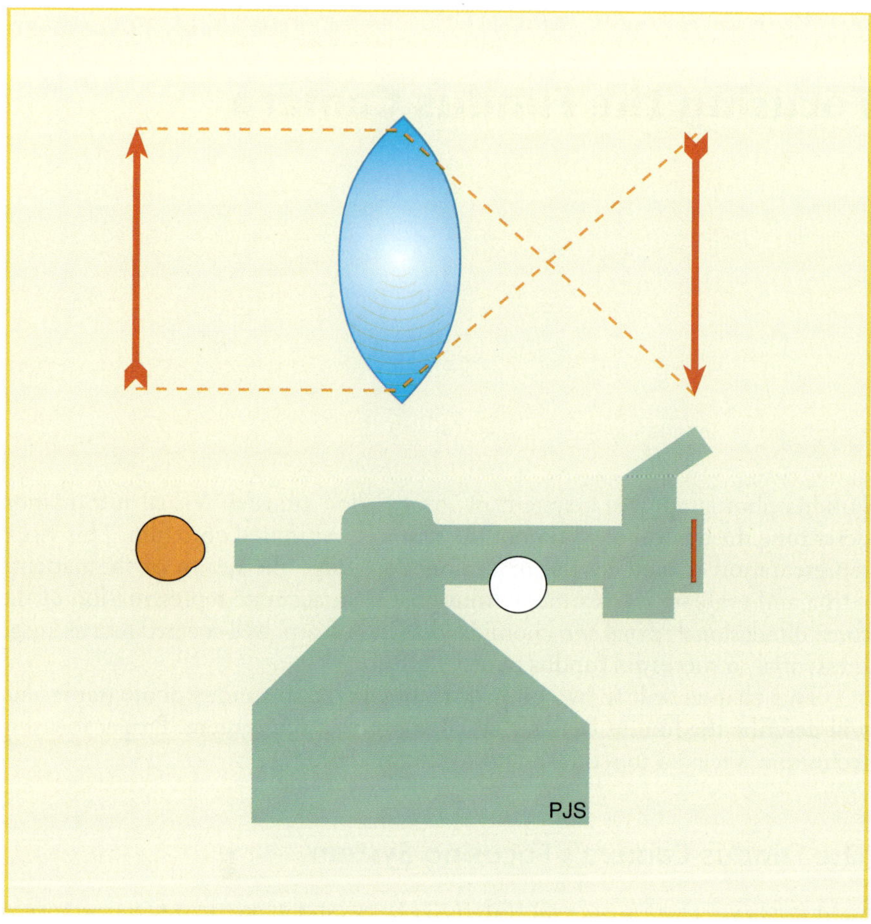

Figure 5–1 ○ A sharp fundus photograph is created when a specific retina layer is the object, the fundus camera optics serve as a lens, and the film plane coincides with the plane of sharp focus.

Single-Lens Reflex Viewing System

The objective lens of the fundus camera transmits light for both viewing the subject and exposing the film (Fig. 5–3). The hinged mirror is positioned differently for viewing and taking the picture. First the image is evaluated through the viewfinder with the mirror in the down position. Then the mirror flips up and out of the way, the shutter opens, the flash is tripped, and the film is exposed to light.

The focusing screen helps the photographer judge image sharpness before exposing the film. The focusing screen and film plane are located equidistant

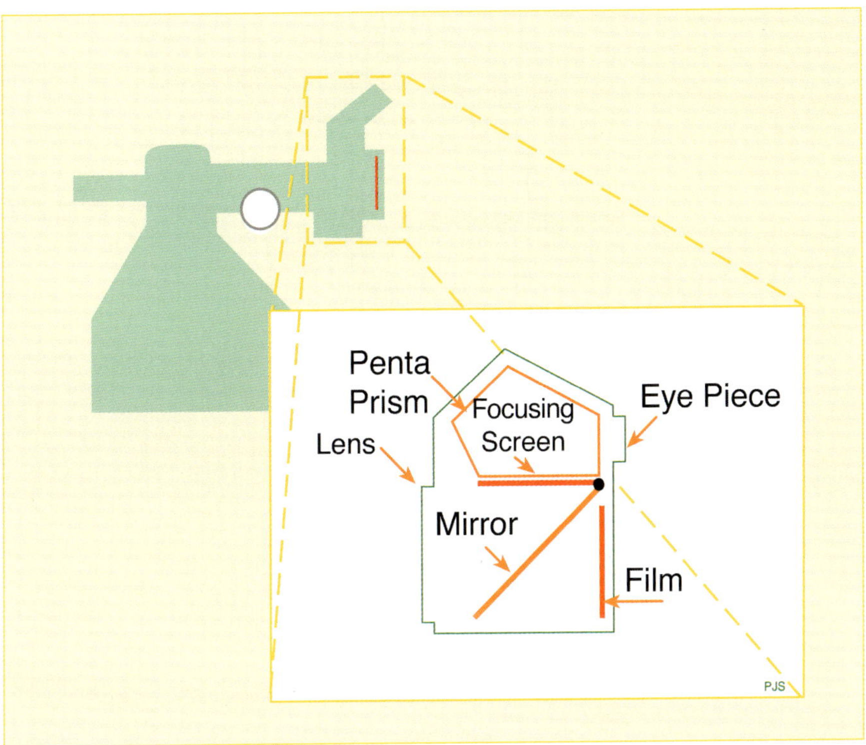

Figure 5–2 ○ Most modern fundus cameras use a single-lens reflex (SLR) system for viewing the fundus image. Standard components of an SLR are identified in this simplified version of the fundus camera's SLR viewing system.

from the objective lens. When an object appears sharp on the focusing screen, its image will also be sharp at the film plane. In standard 35-mm cameras, the focusing screen glass is ground glass either with or without a Fresnel surface.

Light intensity decreases as it is scattered by a standard patterned glass focusing screen, an effect that is of little importance to most photographers. In fundus photography, however, a number of factors make it difficult to use these focusing screens:

1. **Relatively small amounts of light must be used when viewing the eye.** Retinal damage increases as the quantity and duration of illumination increases.[1] Many patients are sensitive to bright lights, making examination with bright light difficult.
2. **High magnifications (e.g., 2.5× in a 30-degree fundus image) are used to photograph the retina.** Light energy from a small portion of the subject

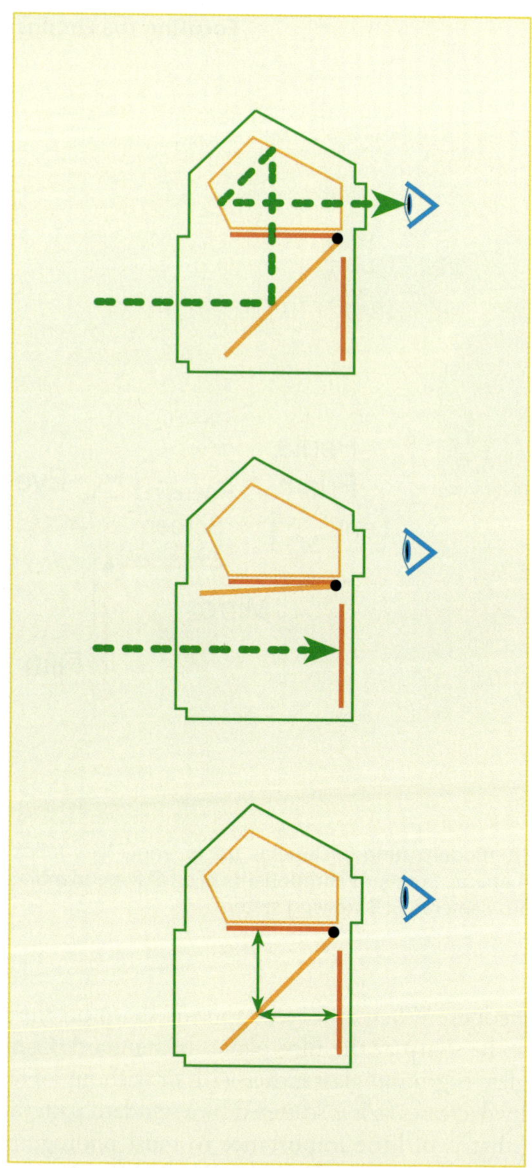

Figure 5–3 ○ Using a single-lens reflex (SLR) camera. When you preview a scene in the viewfinder, the light from the lens enters the camera body and reflects off the hinged, 45-degree mirror (*top*). Your view is the image on the focusing screen. When you choose to expose an image, the mirror flips up and out of the way, momentarily darkening the viewfinder (*center*). This allows the same light that you saw in the viewfinder to expose the film. An SLR system is basically a "what-you-see-is-what-you-get" system. The distance between the focusing screen and the lens system is equal to the distance between the film plane and the lens system (*bottom*). When the image appears sharp on an SLR camera's focusing screen, it will also appear sharp on the film.

is distributed over a physically greater image area when the image is magnified. This results in a relatively lower level of light available for imaging any particular portion of the subject.

3. **The grainy structure of a ground-glass focusing screen breaks up the fine detail of the fundus image.** The relatively large size of the grains in a ground-glass focusing screen make it difficult to focus on the fine retinal details. The main reason for not using ground glass is that it absorbs too much light.

Fundus cameras replace the patterned glass of a standard 35-mm SLR camera system with a clear glass focusing screen containing etched lines (Fig. 5–4). The clear glass maximizes the light entering the photographer's eye. The etched black lines (called the *focusing reticle*) help the photographer to focus on the correct plane.

Because the image in the viewfinder is not "captured" by the focusing screen, but rather floats in the air space both in front of and behind the clear glass, it is termed an *aerial image*. Learning to focus this aerial image by using the reticle is essential to obtaining sharp images with a fundus camera.

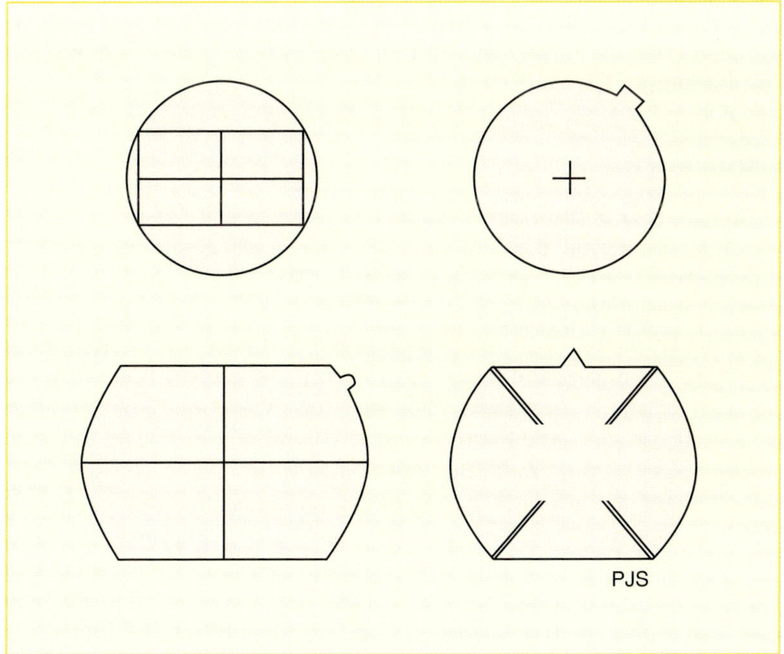

Figure 5–4 ○ Focusing reticles come in various designs that vary according to manufacturer, camera model, and date of manufacture.

Viewing the Aerial Image

When you look through the fundus camera's viewfinder with your best corrected vision, you will see one of four possible views: The image inside the viewfinder may be totally out of focus, without distinct reticle lines or sharp areas of retina; the image alone may be in focus; only the black reticle lines may be in focus; or both the image and the black reticle lines may be in focus. Only in the last case will a sharp retinal image be recorded on film (Fig. 5–5).

If both the focusing reticle and the fundus image are completely out of focus, then one of two conditions may exist. First, your eyes might not be corrected for their best visual acuity. A routine eye examination is recommended when you begin your career and at regular intervals thereafter. Second, the fundus camera's reticle and focus adjustment might be improperly set (see the section below on obtaining a sharp fundus photograph). Of course, a combination of the preceding circumstances may occur.

When you view through a correctly adjusted eyepiece before the fundus has been focused, the retina appears blurry, while the reticle is sharp. Taking a picture will produce an image that is as unsharp as you see it in the viewfinder. After you correctly adjust the eyepiece and the fundus camera's focusing mechanism, both the fundus image and the reticle should be sharp and clear. Your eyes are focused on the reticle, and the image from the fundus camera corresponds with the film plane (Fig. 5–5*H*). Only this final combination yields a sharply focused fundus photograph (Fig. 5–5*I*).

Accommodation

Accommodation is the normal mechanism your eye uses for focusing on near objects. In simple terms, the ciliary muscle tugs or releases tension on the lens zonules, modifying the refractive power of the lens. At the same time, the near reflex causes miosis and convergence. The ability to accommodate lessens with age.

A significant cause of unsharp fundus photographs is accommodation by the photographer during the focusing procedure. When you look through the camera eyepiece and accommodate, you may see a sharp image of the retina but not see a sharp image of the focusing reticle. If you accommodate to perceive a sharp image of the retina, then the optical system of your eye is used to obtain sharpness, rather than the optical system of the fundus camera. You may attempt to sharpen the image using the focusing knob, but a blurry photograph will result.

The tendency to accommodate when focusing is especially prevalent in fatigued or novice fundus photographers and in experienced photographers who are younger than approximately 40 years of age. Strategies for safeguarding against accommodation problems during fundus photography procedures include the following:

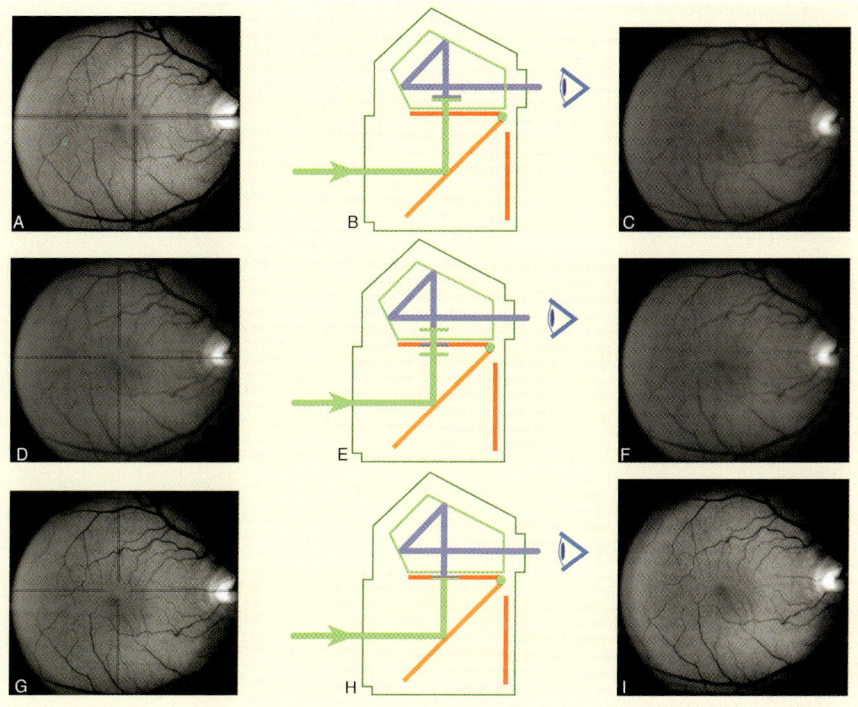

Figure 5–5 ○ Using the reticle to focus. This figure illustrates the relationship between sharpness in the reticle, your fundus view, and the sharpness in the final fundus photograph. When you focus the image without regard to the sharpness of the focusing reticle, you will perceive the fundus image as sharp while the reticle image appears blurry (*A*). The image you see is focused by your eyes above the focusing screen, closer than infinity (*B*). Even though you see a sharp image in the viewfinder, the exposed photograph will be blurry (*C*). When you view through a correctly adjusted eyepiece before the fundus has been focused on, the fundus appears blurry while the reticle is distinctly sharp (*D*). You have correctly focused on the reticle, but the camera's image has not yet been adjusted to coincide with the receiving plane (*E*). If a picture is taken, the resulting image will be as unsharp as you see it in the viewfinder (*F*). After you correctly adjust the eyepiece and the fundus camera's focusing mechanism, both the fundus image and the reticle appear sharp and clear (*G*). Your eyes are focused on the reticle, and the image from the fundus camera corresponds with the film plane (*H*). Only this final combination yields a sharply focused fundus photograph (*I*).

1. Highly trained photographers can feel themselves accommodate. You might want to test this yourself. Find a quiet room with no distractions. Fully relax your mind and body while focusing your eyes on an object at least 20 feet away. Bring your index finger approximately 18 inches from your nose. When you focus on your index finger, notice that the background becomes unsharp. Keeping your finger in focus, move it toward your nose slowly. The background will become increasingly less sharp, and the edges of your visual field will constrict. You will feel your eyes converge, and you might feel a sensation in the anterior section of your eyes. Focus on the distant object again and repeat. With practice, you will become more aware of your personal sensation during accommodation. Awareness of this sensation during fundus photography will alert you to the possibility of accommodation and the unsharp photographs that may result.

2. If you think you are accommodating during a procedure, look away from the eyepiece. Merely blinking or closing your eyes may help to reset their focus. On looking again into the viewfinder, concentrate on the thin black lines of the focusing reticle. Intentionally blurring the fundus image (move the plane of focus into the vitreous by rotating the focusing knob) might help you to concentrate on the reticle image.

3. Try to keep both eyes open throughout the procedure, preferably with the non-eyepiece eye focused across the room. A well-placed visual (of a landscape or distant scene) on the opposite wall of the fundus photography room will promote distance focusing. If the room is especially small, a mirror (or the glass from the above print) may be used to reflect the image from a visual hanging directly behind the photographer. Glancing at this reflection will better approximate distance focusing in a small room. Viewing exciting scenery through a window in a fundus photography room might seem tempting. However, the darkness necessary during procedures precludes this option.

4. A full day of fundus photography can distort the normal accommodative process, causing your eye to be "stuck" in near focus. Accommodative excess is the result of prolonged and intense periods of near work, which may result in eyestrain and headaches.[2,3] Persistent focusing on infinity may help to retard this near-focus spasm. Consciously focus across the distance of the waiting room (or down a long hall) when you call patients. Practice distance focusing out a window during breaks or at lunch. Make a point of looking at distant scenery or buildings while commuting to and from work.

Of course, your eyes should always be corrected to their best visual acuity. You might find that one eye is sharper than the other. Keep your eyeglasses or contact lenses scrupulously clean.

Certain physiologic conditions may also distort the focusing process. Extreme changes in blood sugar may alter the thickness of the diabetic photographer's lens, making distance vision unsharp. Certain drugs may produce pseudopresbyopia.[4] Dry eyes can be a problem if you find yourself blinking less frequently when looking through the fundus camera viewfinder. Use artificial tears or contact lens wetting solution as needed. Maintaining a healthy diet and good physical condition will also help your focusing abilities.

Sharp Fundus Photographs

Definition

Sharpness in a photograph is a visual phenomenon that is difficult to quantify. Both contrast and resolution play a role in our subjective evaluations of sharpness. An image is described as sharp when the borders defining the subject are distinct and clear. An unsharp image contains borders between adjacent areas that are double, overlap, or are difficult to distinguish. A sharp fundus photograph results when the fundus camera's plane of sharp focus coincides with the specific pathology in question.

When photographing the retina, remember that, like most photographic subjects in our three-dimensional world, the posterior segment of the eye has depth. The vitreous, retina, and choroid may be described histologically as overlapping layers of gel, tissue, and blood vessels that are located at specific levels[*] within the eye (Fig. 5–6).

Five distinct levels (the vitreous, inner retina, central retina, outer retina, and choroid) may be distinguished by using white-light, 30-degree stereo fundus photography in many patients with diseased or swollen retinas.

Monochromatic filters (e.g., exciter and barrier filters for fluorescein angiography, blue filters for retinal nerve fiber layer photography, and green filters for "red-free" photography) enhance the photographic separation of retinal levels.[5] Thickened diseased retina, normal-angle fundus camera optics, and stereo imaging also facilitate the recognition of retinal levels and expedite their differential focusing.

Monocular (single-image) photography, wide-angle fundus cameras, and inaccurate focusing inhibit the ability to distinguish five separate retinal levels. The levels' thinness combined with the depth of field of the fundus camera may make it difficult to distinguish each of the five levels in patients with normal or thin retinas.

---

*The term *layer* is used when referring to histologic sections, whereas the term *level* is reserved for discussion of the fundus camera image.

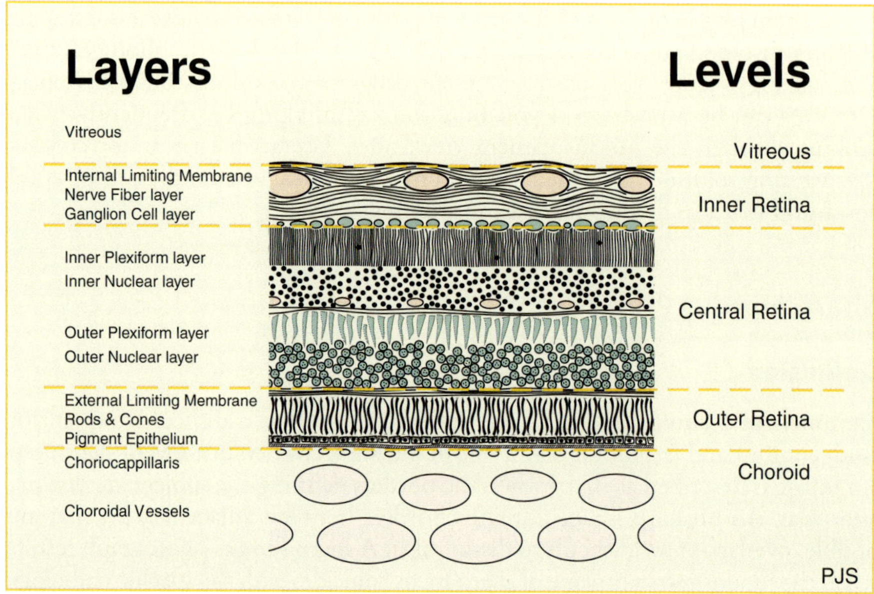

Figure 5–6 ○ Layers and levels. A 10-layer histologic representation of the retina and choroid is related to the five levels that may be distinguished when viewing either a narrow-angle fundus camera viewfinder or the final stereo fundus photograph. Each of these five levels may or may not be able to be distinguished, depending on the thickness and pathology of a particular patient's retina.

A sharp fundus photograph is precisely focused on a specific subject within a specific level of the retina. The objective appearance of clear, distinct borders in a fundus photograph does not in itself certify the sharpness of that photograph. A fundus photograph may be sharp but not at the appropriate retinal level (Fig. 5–7). Focusing too far forward (into the vitreous) or too far back (into the outer retina or choroid) results in a fundus photograph that does not accurately document the pathology of concern.

How can optimal focus at the appropriate layer within the eye be achieved? An understanding of retinal anatomy is essential to achieving sharp fundus photographs.

Retinal Anatomy: Layers and Levels

Accurately adjusting the fundus camera's focus requires an awareness of the layered aspect of the eye's anatomy. The vitreous gel fills the posterior segment of the eye. The retina is a three-dimensional tissue described histologically as 10 separate layers. The choroid contains two layers of blood vessels.

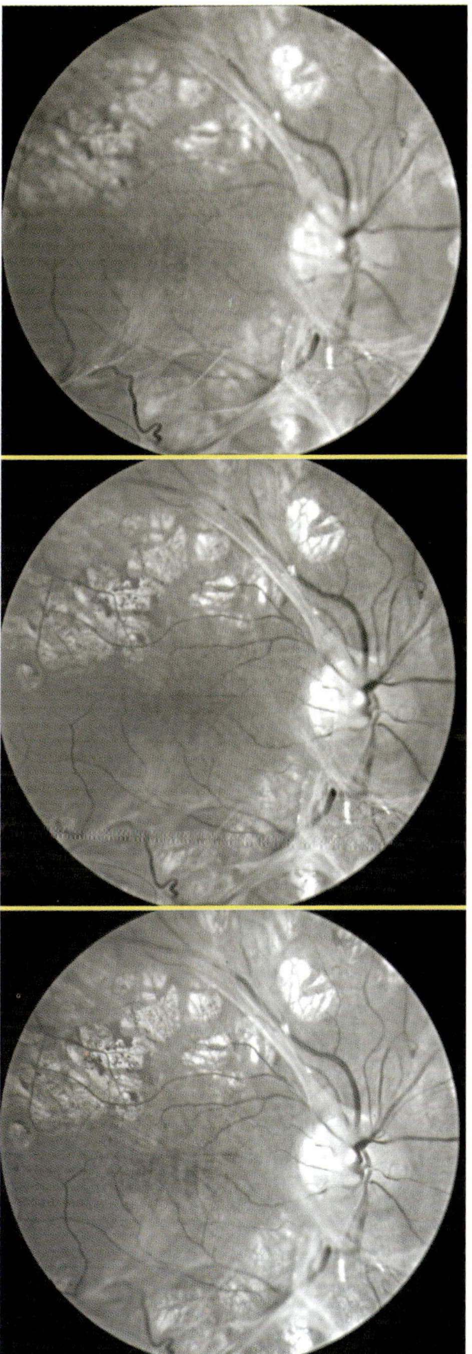

Figure 5–7 ○ This eye was photographed at three different planes of focus. All three images contain areas that may be considered sharp. If the macula is the intended subject of the photograph, however, only the center image can be judged a sharp fundus photograph.

The vitreous is positioned anterior to the retina. In the normal eye, the vitreous cannot be imaged with a standard fundus camera. However, when documentation of a diabetic neovascular frond, a retinal detachment, or asteroid hyalosis is necessary, the fundus camera should be focused "up" into the vitreous, rather than "down" on the retina (Fig. 5–8).

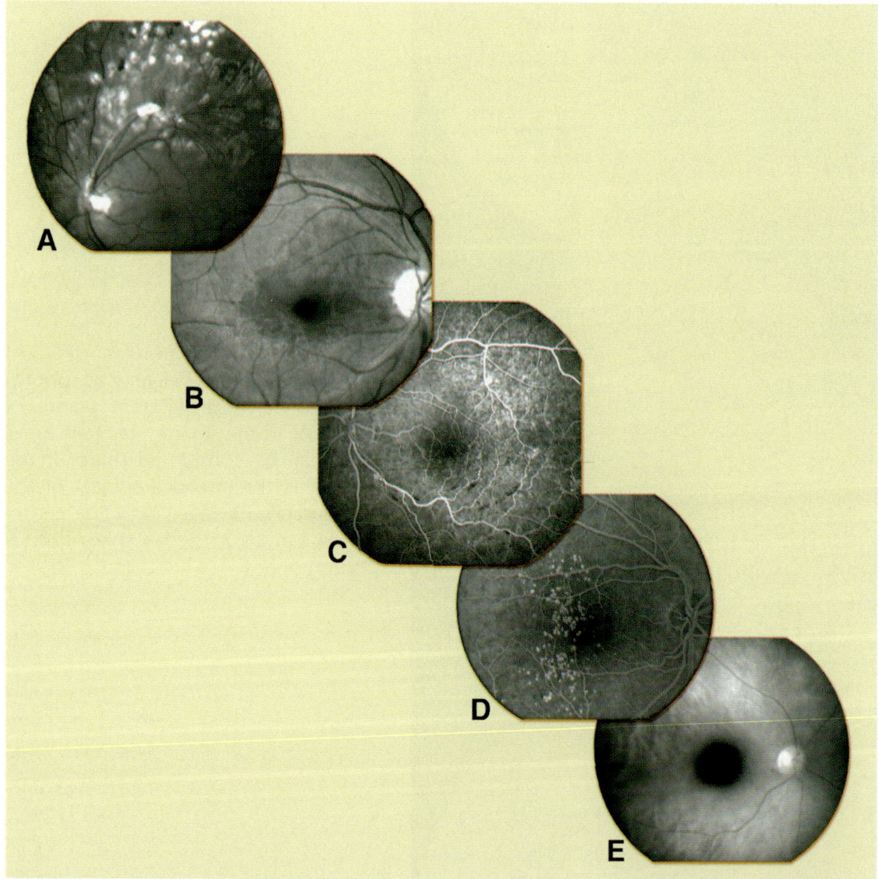

Figure 5–8 ○ Clinical examples of focusing on different levels of the retina are demonstrated in the following images. *A,* Focusing the fundus camera "up" in the vitreous documents neovascularization disc and neovascularization elsewhere. *B,* The nerve fiber layer, accentuated with a blue 490-nm filter, is the object of focus. *C,* The avascular zone surrounding the fovea may be best appreciated when the central portion of the retina is the object of focus. *D,* Focusing on the retinal pigment epithelium or outer retina results in a sharp image of these drusen. *E,* Maximum information at the level of the choroid is achieved through the use of a red (650-nm) filter and careful focusing on the choroidal nevus.

The internal limiting membrane, the nerve fiber layer, and the ganglion cell layer combine to form the inner retina. It is visualized as the nerve fiber layer and the reflections from the large retinal blood vessels. Cotton-wool spots, nerve fiber defects, myelinated nerve fibers, and flame-shaped hemorrhages occur at this level.

The inner and outer plexiform layer and the inner and outer nuclear layer form the central portion of the retina. The central retina contains the smaller blood vessel branches, hard exudates, and diabetic microaneurysms. The capillary net surrounding the foveal avascular zone is imaged during fluorescein angiography when the fundus camera is properly focused on this middle level of the retina.

The outer retinal level includes the rods and cones, the retinal pigment epithelium, and Bruch's membrane. Subretinal neovascular membranes, drusen, presumed ocular histoplasmosis scars, and angioid streaks occur at this level.

The choriocapillaris and major choroidal blood vessels lie below the retina. The surface of nevi and choroidal tumors can be imaged by focusing "down" into the choroid.

Targeting Focus

It is difficult to distinguish 10 different retinal layers when looking through the eyepiece of the fundus camera. However, you can target the focus of the final fundus photograph to a specific level by recognizing its visual contents. Table 5–1 relates common retinal disorders, the affected retinal level, and examples of possible corresponding retinal abnormalities. Targeting focus to a specific level is a matter of recognizing retinal pathology and optimizing the focus to the appropriate retinal depth.

Focusing on the highlights reflected from the large blood vessels results in a sharp photograph of the inner retina. The central retina appears clear in the fundus photograph if the photographer first seeks sharpness in the larger blood vessels, then their branches, and their branches, and so forth. If the granular appearance of the pigment epithelium is focused on, then the outer retina becomes the subject of the photograph. When photographing a subretinal neovascular membrane (located in the outer level of the retina), an unsharp photograph of the offending blood vessels results if you focus on the larger, main retinal blood vessels (found in the inner level of the retina). A sharp image can be obtained by focusing on the drusen that lie directly on the pigment epithelium.

Multiple levels of focus may be chosen in a retina with diabetic macular edema (Fig. 5–9). If you focus on the inner surface of the retina, the photograph will document the elevation of the retina but may render much of the posterior pole blurred. A deeper focus may depict the surface of the swollen macula un-

Table 5–1
Patient Diagnosis and Retinal Levels

Patient's Diagnosis	Examples of Possible Abnormalities	Retinal Level
Asteroid hyalosis	Lipid deposits	Vitreous
Diabetic retinopathy	Neovascular fronds	
Retinoschisis	Elevated retinal sensory layers	
Retinal detachment	Elevated retina	
Diabetic retinopathy	Cotton-wool spots	Inner retina
Glaucoma	Nerve fiber layer defects, optic disc borders	
Hypertensive retinopathy	Cotton-wool spots	
Macular hole	Edges of macular hole	
Preretinal membrane	Cellophane maculopathy	
Retinal hemorrhage	Preretinal hemorrhage, subhyaloid hemorrhage	
Retinal vein occlusion	Flame-shaped hemorrhages	
Cystoid macular edema	Swelling	Central retina
Diabetic retinopathy	Microaneurysms, hard exudates, dot and blot hemorrhages, macular edema	
Retinal artery occlusion	Blocked artery	
Retinal vein occlusion	Neovascularization	
Retinitis pigmentosa	Bone-spicule-like pigment	
Age-related macular degeneration	Subretinal neovascular membranes, drusen	Outer retina
Central serous retinopathy	Pigment epithelium defect	
Hereditary abnormalities	Angioid streaks	
Presumed ocular histoplasmosis syndrome	Subretinal neovascular membranes, punched out hypopigmented areas	
AMPPE	Choroidal disturbance	Choroid
Nevus	Surface texture	
Optic nerve head drusen	Drusen under disc	
Choroidal tumor	Surface texture	

AMPPE = acute multifocal placoid pigment epitheliopathy.
Note: Sample patient diagnoses are listed and related to the retinal layers that are visible through the fundus camera. Examples of possible retinal abnormalities (which may or may not be evident in each specific patient) are correlated. To target the focus to a specific layer, note the patient's diagnosis, and focus on the specific abnormalities. If the retina is abnormally thick, you might be able to focus on the same retinal field at different levels. Double-check the focus with each field change.

sharply but will clearly reveal any hard exudates, blot hemorrhages, or both. Focusing in the central retina will accurately document the leaking retinal blood vessels in a fluorescein angiogram.

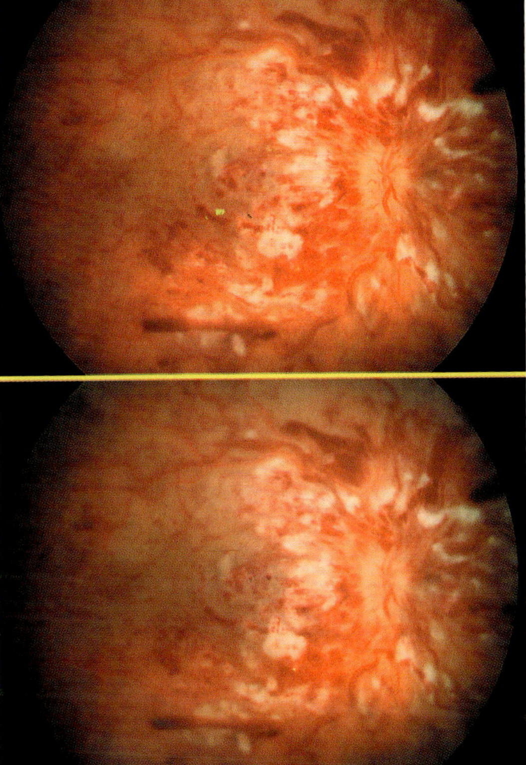

Figure 5–9 ○ With significant retinal elevation, should you focus on the highest elevation (*bottom*) or the general level of the retina (*top*)? Use your professional judgment, or expose multiple photographs.

The fundus camera's depth of field is a focusing consideration. In focusing a fundus camera, only the single level that has been targeted will be in critically sharp focus. When the final photograph is viewed, however, more than one level may appear acceptably sharp. This range of acceptably sharp focus extends both in front of and behind the actual plane of sharp focus.

Wide-angle fundus cameras produce a greater depth of field than do normal-angle cameras if the same eye is photographed and the exposed film area is identical (Fig. 5–10). It is not the angle of the optics but rather the decrease in magnification that contributes to the increased impression of sharpness.[6]

A working knowledge of depth of field helps in documenting the retina. Focusing on the central retina (in a normal, clear eye) yields a final photograph in which the outer retina and possibly the inner retina are acceptably sharp. However, if you focus on the granular appearance of the retinal pigment epithelium, then the inner retina will most likely not be in sharp focus.

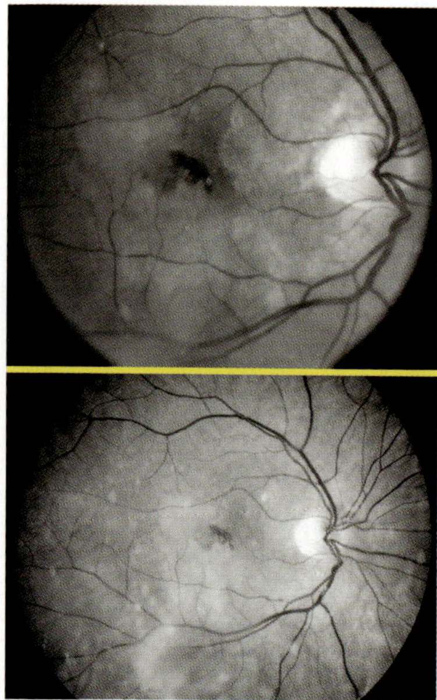

Figure 5–10 ○ When narrow-angle (*top*) and wide-angle (*bottom*) photographs of this eye with asteroid hyalosis are compared, the wide-angle image appears to have greater depth of field because of its smaller magnification.

Depth of focus is found at the film plane and usually mirrors the depth of field located at the subject plane. The depth of focus in most traditional imaging systems is relatively flat. This corresponds with the flatness of the film that is used as a receiving plane (Fig. 5–11). The depth of field in most fundus camera lens systems is curved to mimic the shape of the normal retina. In well-corrected fundus camera optical systems, the curved plane of the subject's detail is translated into a flat plane to match the film plane. In less well-corrected fundus camera lens systems, the plane of the depth of focus is just as curved as the depth of field. Fundus cameras that exhibit this curved depth of focus yield film images that are unsharp at the edges when the camera is focused centrally (and are unsharp centrally when focused on the edges). The intended subject will appear sharp on the film only with careful composition and focus.

Sharpness Limitations of the Camera

The sharpness of a final fundus photograph is, of course, limited by the sharpness of the specific camera's optical system. Objective tests comparing the relative sharpness of various fundus cameras are unavailable. However, experience with multiple cameras in a clinical setting has yielded some general guidelines.

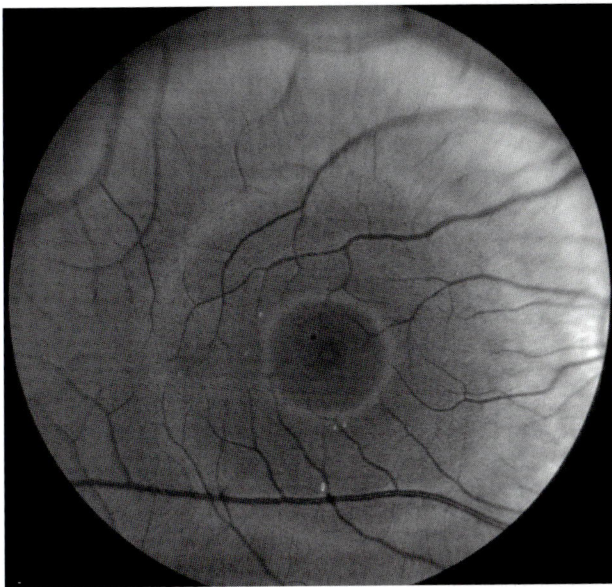

Figure 5–11 ○ Images from a well-corrected fundus camera closely match the curvature of the retina. Learn the limitations of your particular camera by carefully focusing on the fovea of a clear eye and then evaluating the actual sharpness at the edges of the processed photograph.

Resolution of fine detail decreases as the magnification decreases because less film area is used for creating an image of a particular detail. When two fundus cameras have imaging circles of equal size, the wide-angle fundus camera (greater than 45 degrees) will be less able to resolve fine detail than the normal-angle camera (30 degrees). When two fundus cameras have optics of equal quality, the fundus camera with higher magnification will achieve better definition of fine retinal details.

Resolution and contrast decrease with the introduction of angle-changing lens systems (Fig. 5–12). Multiple-angle cameras typically have one best setting—often the widest angle. An optical departure from this angle of view degrades image quality. However, greater magnification may yield details that are not perceived under low magnification (Fig. 5–13). Use your professional judgment to determine the most appropriate angle of view for a specific fundus photograph, or expose multiple images for later editing.

Wide-angle cameras suffer greater losses in resolution from local areas of potential blurriness (e.g., a cataract or a corneal scar) than do normal-angle

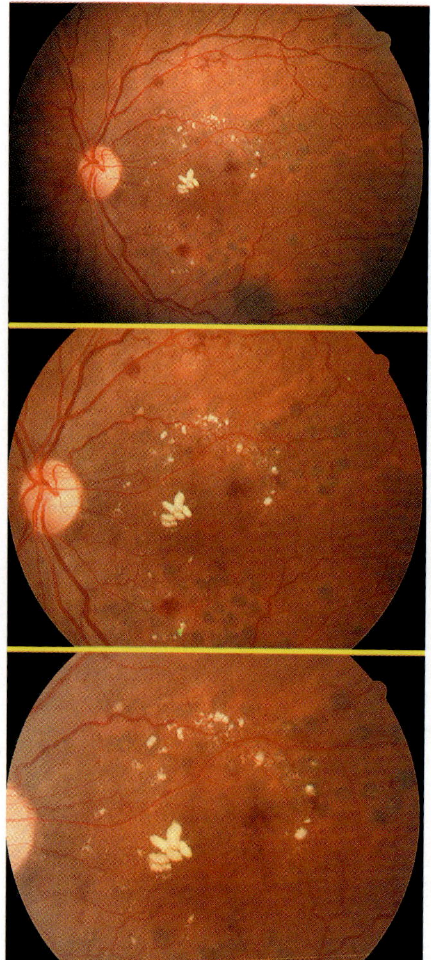

Figure 5–12 ○ Carefully focus and photograph a sampling of clear-eyed patients with each angle of view. Examine the images together to discern the sharpness and contrast characteristics of each angle choice.

cameras. This phenomenon is due to the larger bundle of returning image-forming rays that constitute the wide-angle image. The thinner bundles of normal-angle camera optics are more likely to permit you to select small pockets of clear media.

Remember that newer fundus cameras of the same design may be sharper than older cameras and that "identical" cameras of the same design and vintage may produce images with slightly different results.

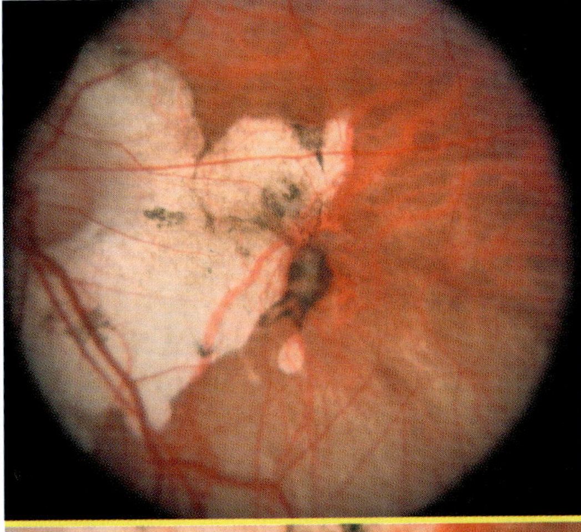

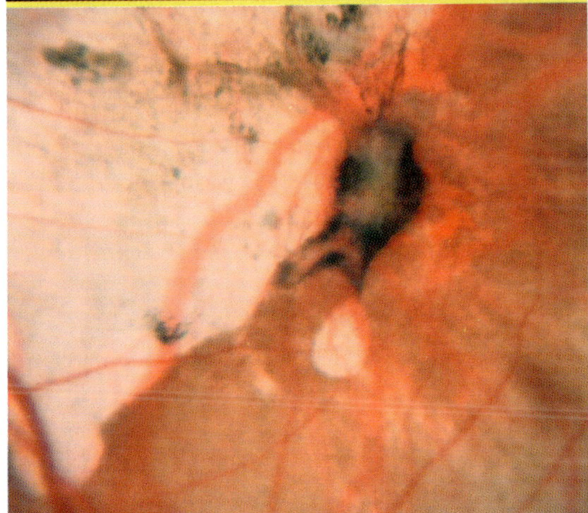

Figure 5–13 ○ Although the sharpness and contrast of magnified images (*bottom*) may be compromised, they often provide useful information.

A fundus camera's cost is not directly proportional to the sharpness of its optics. Lens performance, cost, and ease of use must each be considered separately. Although a low price and ergonomic design should be considered when purchasing a fundus camera, actual lens performance is critical.

Only the publication of unbiased data detailing the actual performance of many different fundus cameras allows fair comparisons to be made. Until such tests are designed and implemented, the opinions of other ophthalmic photographers and personal experience must guide us.[7]

Focusing Technique

If you conscientiously use the reticle and practice a deliberate focusing procedure, you will produce consistently sharp fundus photographs. The eyepiece must be correctly set to obtain a sharp view of the reticle. Instructions for adjusting the eyepiece are found in the sidebar on setting your reticle. A suggested focusing procedure is as follows:

1. Review the patient's photograph request form and prior photographs. Note the working diagnosis.
2. Seat the patient at the instrument, and explain the procedure.
3. Adjust the headrest, chinrest, joystick, and camera head height while looking around the side of the camera. Align the patient and camera so that the retina and the film plane are parallel. Project the doughnut of light into the center of the dilated pupil. Position the illumination system by obtaining a sharp image of the viewing light's filament on the cornea or closed outer eyelid.
4. Turn off the room lights. Your view through the viewfinder will brighten, and your eye's depth of field will decrease as a result of your slightly dilated pupils. It will be easier for you to discriminate between retinal layers with this shallower depth of field. In addition, the darkened room enhances the figure-ground relationship between the external fixation light and its background. This allows the patient to follow the external fixation device more easily.
5. Establish patient fixation. (Focusing on a moving target is difficult.)
6. Look through the ocular, and visualize the focusing reticle. Constant awareness of this reticle throughout the focusing procedure is necessary for obtaining sharp fundus photographs. Dust specks may be visible in the viewfinder. If these dust specks are on the same plane as the etched lines, use them like the reticle. If you are unsure of their precise location, consult a knowledgeable service technician to either clean the dust specks or determine the specific plane on which they rest.
7. Adjust the image for maximum color saturation and minimum artifacts. Move the fixation light to visualize the requested retinal field.
8. Begin turning the focusing knob. You will see the retinal image begin to sharpen. Check the sharpness of the focusing reticle, and decide on which retinal level to focus. Myopic, hyperopic, and aphakic patients may require that you adjust the compensation lens system (diopter control). Myopic patients (long axial length) may need a minus diopter compensation. Hyperopic patients (short axial length) and patients without their natural lenses may require a plus diopter correction. A small black antireflection dot in the front element may be imaged by some cameras when patients

with high myopia are photographed. Both this artifact and the use of the diopter compensation lens system can be eliminated by requesting highly myopic patients to wear their contact lenses while being photographed.[8]

9. As the plane of sharpness travels inward with the rotation of the focusing knob, the vitreous, inner retina, central retina, outer retina, and finally choroidal levels will become sharp in turn. The focusing reticle must always remain sharp.

10. Stop focusing inward as the targeted level is passed and becomes unsharp again.

11. "Rock" the focus (with tiny forward and backward movements of the focusing knob) until the sharpest focus has been obtained. Recheck the sharpness of the focusing reticle.

12. Patient fixation or camera position is adjusted until the precise field of view is obtained. Recheck crosshair sharpness and retinal focus. The area of primary importance should be photographed first, as the best images are often obtained at the beginning of the photo session when both you and the patient are fresh. Many patients require photographs of both the macula and the disc. Focusing on the macula first will approximate more closely the general depth of the retina.

13. Evaluate the need for the astigmatism control (if available). If the image of the fundus seems not quite sharp or if the blood vessels appear elongated in a single direction, then adjusting the astigmatism control may be useful (Fig. 5–14). Sharp posterior pole photographs of patients with keratoconus and patients with large amounts of corneal astigmatism and peripheral photography may require astigmatic correction. Imaging rays traverse an oblique cross section of the lens and cornea in peripheral fundus photography, creating an image that may appear smeared or stretched in a single direction.

14. Constantly monitor the focus throughout the procedure. Recheck the focus each time you change fields; a diseased retina may or may not be elevated in different areas (Fig. 5–15). Monitor the focus during side-to-side changes in camera position during stereo photography. Peripheral fundus photography necessitates a change in the camera-cornea distance and will require focus adjustment. The axial length of most patients' eyes varies slightly from right to left. If alternating photographs of the right and left eye are required and a large focusing discrepancy exists between the two eyes (e.g., OD aphakic, OS intraocular lens), then a small piece of tape on the right and left focusing knobs may be used to mark each side's correct adjustment.[9] Although these landmarks will help you to adjust the camera more quickly as the alternate eyes are photographed, always check your viewfinder for a final focus.

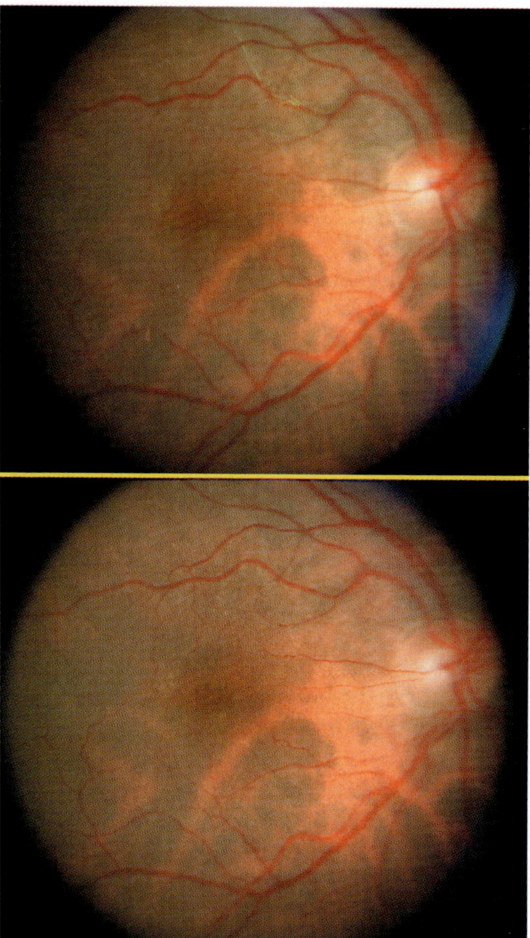

Figure 5–14 ○ If the fundus looks stretched or just slightly out of focus, consider using the astigmatic compensation knob. This control is useful for patients who have large amounts of astigmatism (e.g., after surgery) or in photographing the periphery. Seek your best focus (*top*), and then visually determine whether rotating the knob will be beneficial (*bottom*).

Assuming a par-focal digital/film system, red-free photographs may be used to obtain instant feedback as to focusing accuracy.

Focusing is an acquired skill that requires both practice and a keen understanding of the retinal landscape. Constant awareness of the focusing reticle and precisely targeting the focus to a specific retinal level are keys to success.

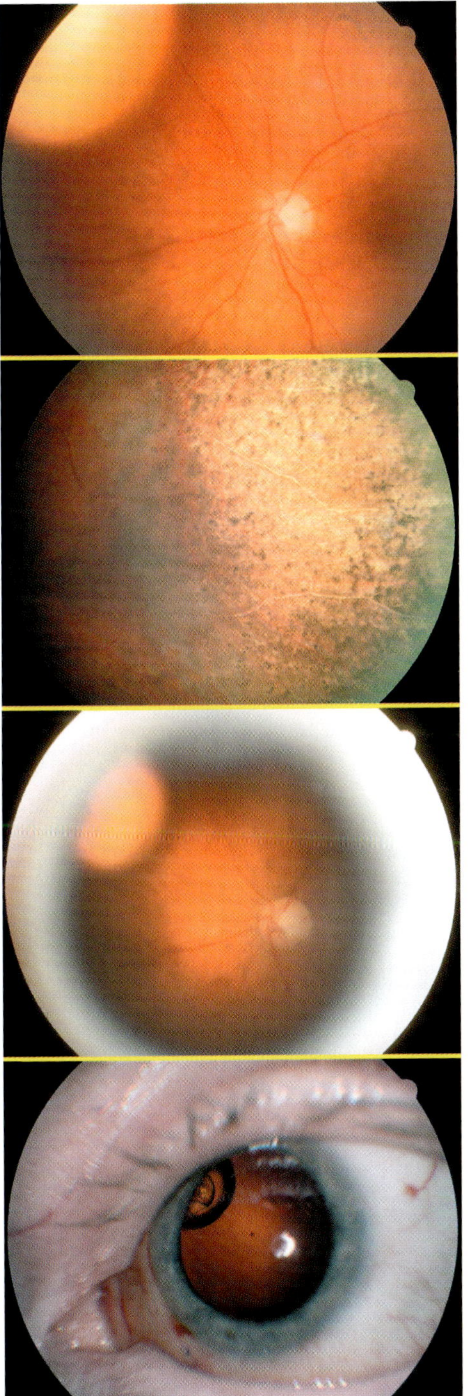

Figure 5–15 ○ Be prepared to alter your focus or alignment to capture items of interest extending into the vitreous. As the camera is pulled back, the yellow artifact in this posterior pole photograph (*top*) of a patient with cytomegalovirus retinitis (*second*) is revealed to be a ganciclovir implant (*third, bottom*).

References

1. Fishman M, Waxler M, Sliney DH, et al.: Symposium on light toxicity and its meaning to ophthalmic photographers. J Ophthalmol Photog 1987;10:6.
2. Holladay JT: Optics, Refraction, and Contact Lenses: Basic and Clinical Science Course. San Francisco: American Academy of Ophthalmology, 1988, p. 173.
3. Milder B, Rubin M: The Fine Art of Prescribing Glasses Without Making a Spectacle of Yourself. Gainesville, FL: Triad Scientific Publishers, 1978, p. 27.
4. Holladay JT: Optics, Refraction, and Contact Lenses: Basic and Clinical Science Course. San Francisco: American Academy of Ophthalmology, 1988, p. 109.
5. Ducrey NM, Delori FC, Gragoudas ES: Monochromatic ophthalmoscopy and fundus photography. Arch Ophthalmol 1979;97:288.
6. Blaker A: Handbook for Scientific Photography. San Francisco: W.H. Freeman, 1977, p. 97.
7. George TW, D'Anna SA: Comparison of retinal fundus cameras: User's survey results. Ophthalmology Instrument and Book Supplement 1983;90(Suppl):80.
8. Kelly MP: A superior method of achieving high myopic retinal focus. J Ophthalmol Photog 1995;17:66.
9. Schatz H, Burton T, Yannuzzi L, Rabb M: Interpretation of fundus fluorescein angiography. St. Louis: Mosby, 1978, p. 27.

Chapter 6

Stereo Fundus Photography

The ophthalmic photographer's ability to record accurate three-dimensional fundus images is one of the most exciting capabilities in our profession. Stereo fundus photography permits clinical examination of the patient's pathology beyond the ordinary two-dimensional view of a conventional photograph. It is fascinating to be able to study an image of an optic nerve, diabetic hemorrhages, vascular occlusion, a macular hole, or a tumor without patient movement and in three dimensions!

Stereopsis (from the Greek word *stereos*, meaning "solid," hence "solid vision") is the ability of the brain to reconstruct a true sense of depth from the flat images transmitted from the two eyes.

The eye, not unlike a camera, is equipped to focus light rays on a light-sensitive substrate. The retina plays the role of the film and is responsible for mapping the formed images. Otherwise, the dynamic, interactive characteristics of the living eye, coupled with the complexities of retinal and cortical visual processing, give results that are quite different from the static interpretation offered by even the finest cameras. Even so, the retina and photographic film have a common limitation: They can provide only a two-dimensional map of the three-dimensional world. Photographers, artists, and one-eyed people will be quick to add that many depth clues are encoded in a single, flat image, but the most immediate and elaborate sense of depth requires not only images from two different vantage points (i.e., two eyes), but also the neural processing that produces stereopsis.

In stereo fundus photography, two slightly different images are created photographically and, when viewed, are fused by the brain. When you view the images, your left eye is presented with the left image, your right eye is presented with the right image, and your brain then recreates the depth relationships that were observed at the time of photography (Fig. 6–1). If you have created the

97

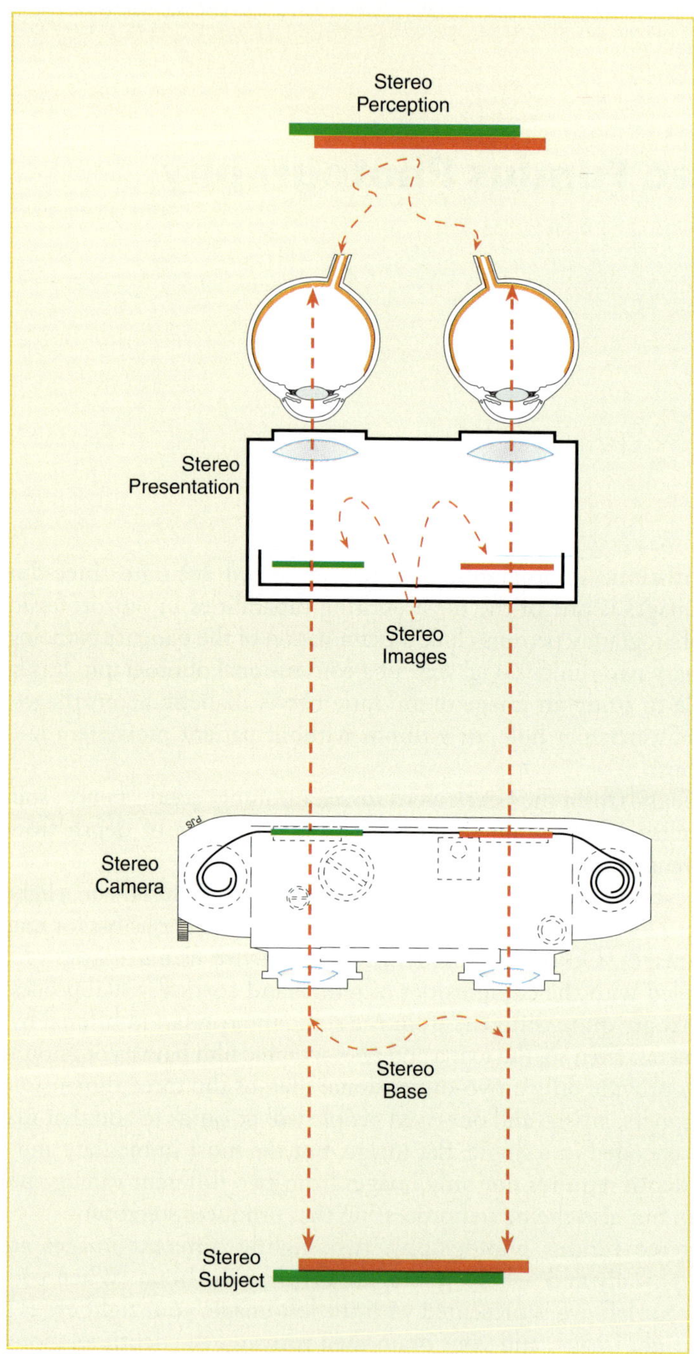

Figure 6–1 ○ Conventional stereo photographic technique has all of the optics and imaging planes parallel to the subject. The stereo base, the separation between the optics, is held constant throughout the optical system.

stereo photographs by a reproducible technique, they may also permit comparison of three-dimensional changes over time.

Many ophthalmologic photographers routinely expose all fundus images in stereo. Obtaining two exposures is a good idea in case a single image is not perfect. Why not provide extra information by taking them as a stereo pair? Accept the challenge: Photograph every fundus in stereo, and you will find—literally—a new dimension in fundus photography.

Terminology note: The phrases that are used to describe a stereo image can be confusing. At times, a "stereo pair" is used to discuss two images that make up a stereo image, whereas at other times you will see "a single stereo image" used to discuss the two images that make up the "stereo pair." Thus, though it might seem a bit confusing, "stereo pair" and "a (single) stereo image" mean the same thing.

Instrumentation and Technique

The technique used in fundus photography takes advantage of the smallness of the subject, the flatness of the subject, the lack of a distant subject, and, most important, the anatomy of the normal human eye.

Most modern mydriatic fundus cameras are capable of producing sequential stereo images—that is, taking one image of a stereo pair and then the other. Precise techniques are needed to create clinical image pairs of the highest quality with the least stress to the patient.

This close-up macro-photography technique is easily accomplished by using the optics of the human eye. The requirements for camera positioning are evaluated from the perspective of the optical systems that are in front of the retina—that is, the cornea and lens.

Understanding the optical systems makes it easier for the photographer to achieve consistent stereo images. Light rays traced from a single point on the human fundus are imaged by the eye's optical components at a distant point, perhaps even at infinity (Fig. 6–2). Convergence (rotation of the camera viewpoint) occurs inside the patient's eye because the optics of the eye is being used in taking the fundus photographs. It is this phenomenon that permits corneal-induced parallax stereo photography to image the same point of the fundus from two vantage points.

The Allen Stereo Technique, described in 1964 by Lee Allen, is used for sequential stereo fundus photographs. Positioning of the camera for stereo fundus photography starts in the same manner as for monocular fundus photography. The camera is shifted first slightly to the left and then to the right of the central position, the stereo pair being thus exposed at each position (Fig. 6–3).

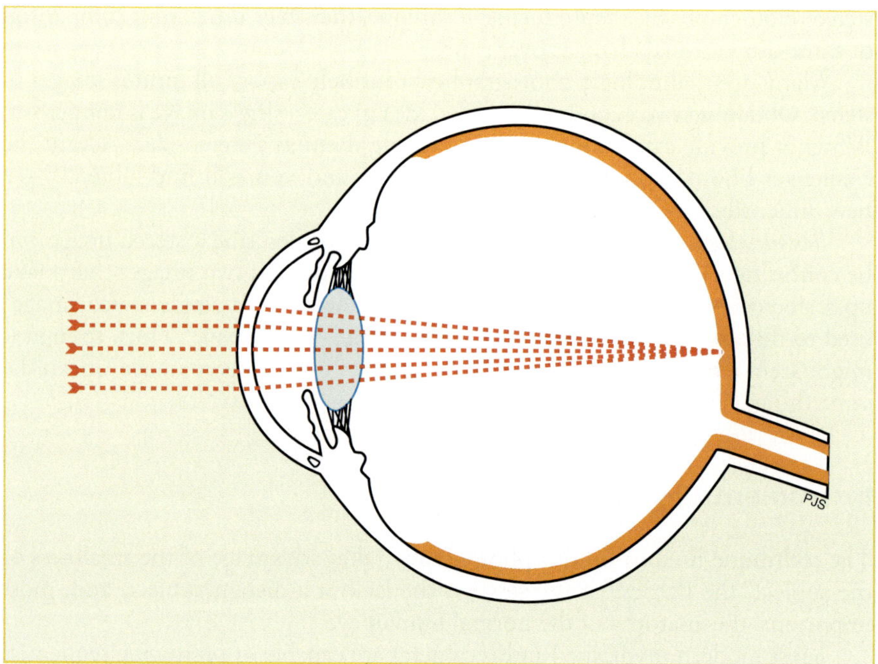

Figure 6–2 ○ The eye in cross section showing parallel light (infinity) converging on a single point on the fundus. Imaging rays coming from the patient's fundus also produces similar parallel rays of light. A fundus camera pointed at any portion of the pupil records an image of the same part of the fundus. Sliding the camera simply records the fundus from a different vantage point.

The stereo base, the distance that the fundus camera lens is moved laterally, defines the amount of stereopsis: the three-dimensional effect. The greater the stereo base is, the greater is the stereo depth effect. If the image is taken with a wide-field fundus camera, the lower image magnification will decrease the apparent depth effect.[1]

Simultaneous stereo cameras (Fig. 6–4) have the distinct advantage of providing the physician with images that are guaranteed to be of constant stereo base, although not necessarily the same position.[2] This technique allows both subjective and analytical analysis to be made with a greater degree of accuracy, as the stereo photographs are exposed with an identical image magnification and stereo base at the exact same moment in time.

Photographing stereo images simultaneously offers additional advantages. Patient cooperation is not needed while two photographs are taken, and there is only one flash for each stereo pair of images. The disadvantage is the difficulty of

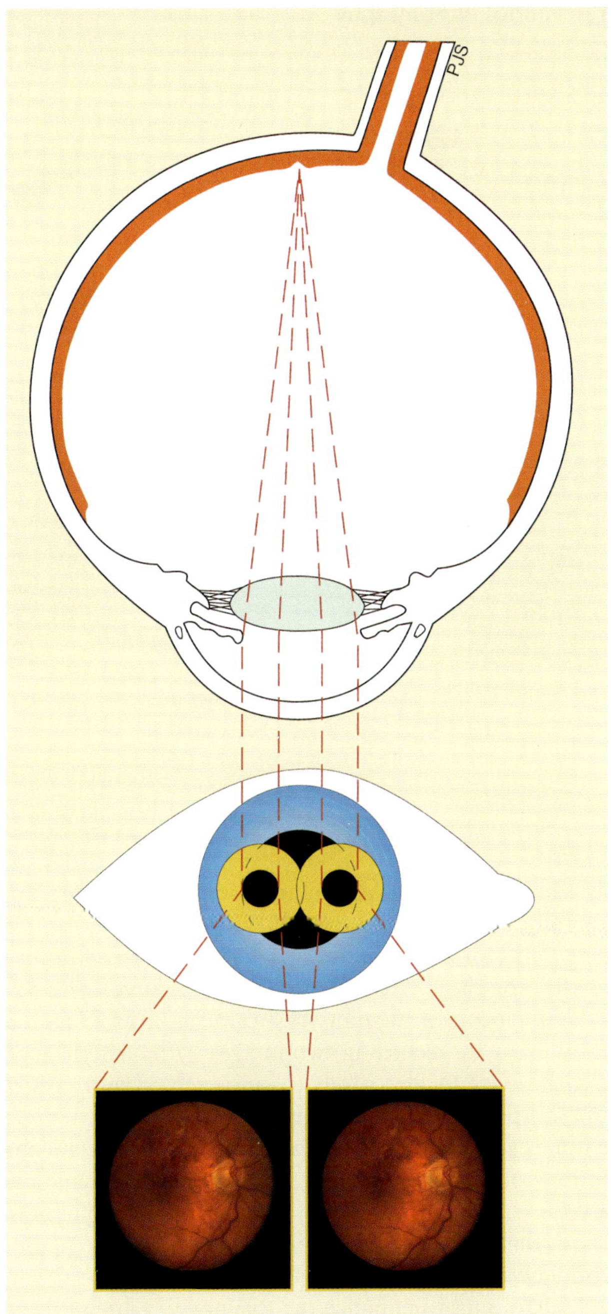

Figure 6–3 ○ Stereo fundus imaging. Two fundus photographs are required to make a stereo pair. The diagram shows the pupillary positioning of the two image areas (*small dark circles*) and the fundus camera's doughnut of illuminating light for stereo fundus photography.

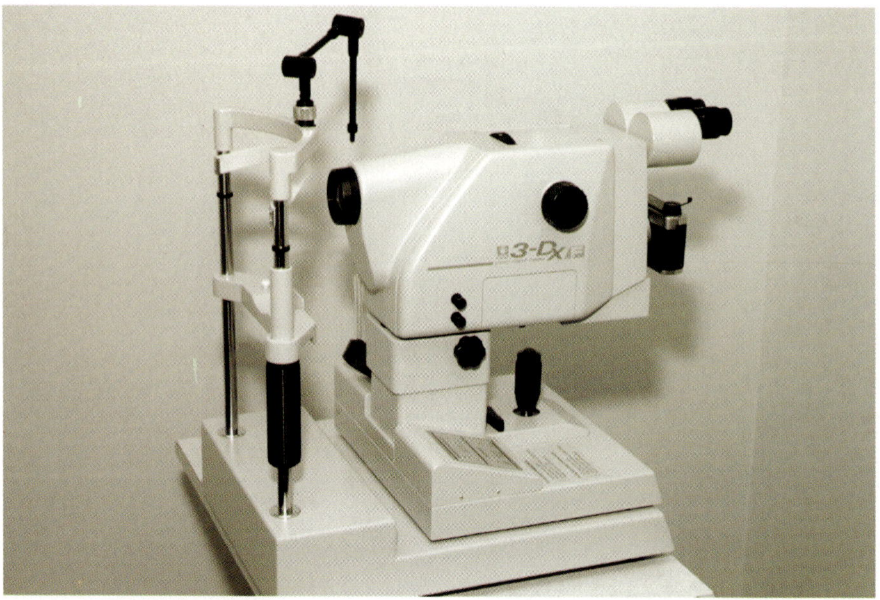

Figure 6–4 ○ The Nidex 3Dx, an example of a simultaneous stereo fundus camera.

simultaneously finding two clear, sharp, and evenly illuminated images through the same potentially small pupil.

The starting point for alignment of simultaneous stereo fundus photography is the same as that for monocular photography; however, you must have two images aligned simultaneously. Aligning these cameras properly requires a modified technique because you are recording two images with a single exposure. Check the quality of each image by alternately closing each of your eyes to ensure that both images are sharp and evenly illuminated.

Once the film is processed and returned, it is very important that you review your work. During camera alignment and photography, the brain does a marvelous job of registering even a marginal stereo image, and you may be astonished to find, on occasion, that one-half of your image pair is of low quality. Constantly check your work and refine your technique.

Specialized techniques to enhance the diagnostic value of the stereo images include differential focusing for stereo imaging and vertical stereo to increase the three-dimensional information of lesions that are better seen with the stereo base in a vertical plane.[2]

Working with Stereo Images

Once stereo images have been exposed and processed, they are prepared for viewing. This section describes how stereo image pairs are identified and how they are mounted and labeled for viewing.

Selecting only the best-quality images of each view helps to maintain a medical record of the highest quality. This is easier when stereo images are photographed using a standard sequence. The photographer should check all processed stereo images to ensure that they are properly aligned and that the stereo-depth relationships are correct. Ensure that the retinal blood vessels are seen in front of the choroid and that optic nerve cupping is seen as a depression, not as an elevation. It is important to be familiar with normal and abnormal retinal pathology, because it is relatively easy to trick an inexperienced viewer into perceiving a depression where there is in fact an elevation or vice versa. Only the best pairs should be saved and labeled as stereo. The slides can simply be placed in a standard slide page with the stereo images paired together. Monocular images may also be kept but not marked as stereo.

A conventional 35-mm transparency in a 2×2 slide mount is the most common film format. Except for photographic competition entries and specially designed stereo projection systems, we suggest using 2×2 mounts to store, view, and project your clinical stereo slides. This choice permits the easy projection of a single monocular frame for conventional (nonstereo) projection (Fig. 6–5).

Split-frame 35-mm slides are "ready-to-go" stereo pairs. The easiest filing solution is to use split-frame stereo pairs mounted in conventional 2×2 slide mounts. Make sure that the film-processing laboratory understands that these are stereo images and that two similar images are to be mounted in one standard mount. Occasionally, a laboratory will mount 36 stereo images as 72 half-frame 2×2 slide mounts. To avoid confusion, send a correctly mounted sample slide or an explanatory note with the unprocessed film.

Marking of the stereo pairs can be accomplished by using a variety of methods. Pairs for a particular patient from each visit can be numbered sequentially and identified as to whether the individual image is the left or the right image

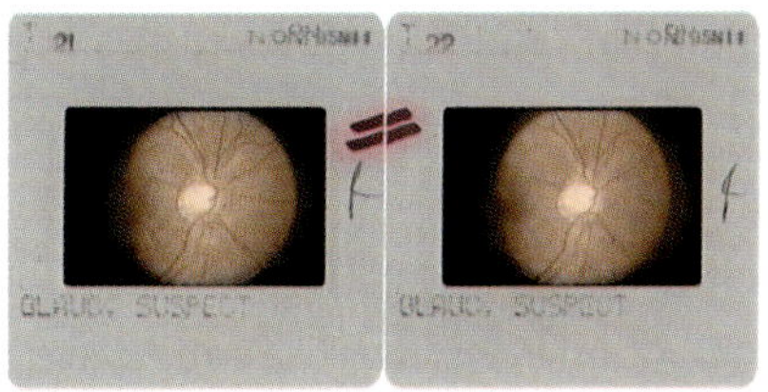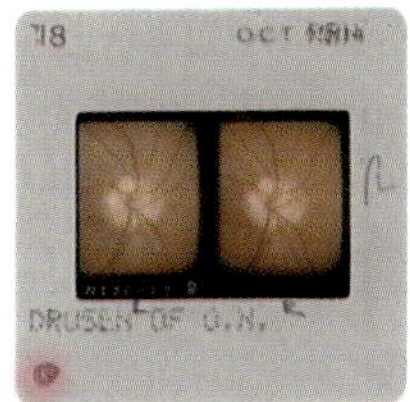

Figure 6–5 ○ Stereo slide formats. *Left,* Two 2×2 35-mm slides. *Right,* Split-frame 35-mm slide mount.

(Fig. 6–6). If the slides are not to be removed from the plastic slide pages, then a simple line or a pair of lines may be used to indicate stereo pairs, or the word "stereo" can be written or rubber-stamped between the two slides.[3]

Viewing Stereo Images

Personal viewing techniques fall into two categories based on image size: images that are smaller and images that are larger than the average pupillary distance of approximately 60 mm.[4] Of the two techniques that allow you to perceive stereo images without viewing paraphernalia, one requires that you accommodate your focus but not to converge your eyes, called *parallel viewing*, and the other requires that you overconverge your eyes (cross-eye) to achieve stereopsis. All other techniques require optical devices to assist you in seeing the stereo images.

The most commonly used stereo viewing techniques in ophthalmology utilize two full-frame, 35-mm stereo slides. The slide that is exposed through the left side of the pupil is positioned in the viewer so that it is viewed by your left eye, and the right image is positioned so that it can be viewed by your right eye. Most stereo slide viewers contain a pair of +4D to +12D lenses (Fig. 6–7). This permits you to relax your accommodation and avoid convergence. The best stereo viewers use compound lenses to reduce distortion and increase sharpness. Once the two images are seen as one, you can adjust the focus either with a focusing adjustment or by physically changing the distance between the slides and the lenses. For extensive viewing, you might consider having an optical shop make you some +8 to +10 glasses.[5]

If you have a large amount of accommodation or are myopic, or both, you might not need a viewer. Simply place the slides side by side (or with a space between the slide mounts up to 10 mm) on a light table, and orient your eyes exactly perpendicular to the center of the slides. Using a sloping light box may make it easier to position your head and eyes properly. Place your face very close to the slides, and relax your convergence by imagining that you are looking far into space. Allow both images to overlap and then become one image. Do not be concerned about image sharpness at this point. Rather, keep your eyes perpendicular to the two slides, and slowly move your head away from the slides to a distance of 6–8 inches while attempting to focus on the slides without losing the single image and having it become two images. If you see two separate images, you are moving back from the slides too quickly, and your eyes are converging. Relax and try again. Viewing stereo slides cannot be practiced in a rush. With practice, you may be able to grab a slide page out of a chart, hold it up to a light source, and view the images in stereo. The key phrase is "with practice."

Split-frame (sometimes mistakenly called *half-frame*) stereo images have two vertical images displayed on a single 35-mm slide frame (Fig. 6–8). Most camera

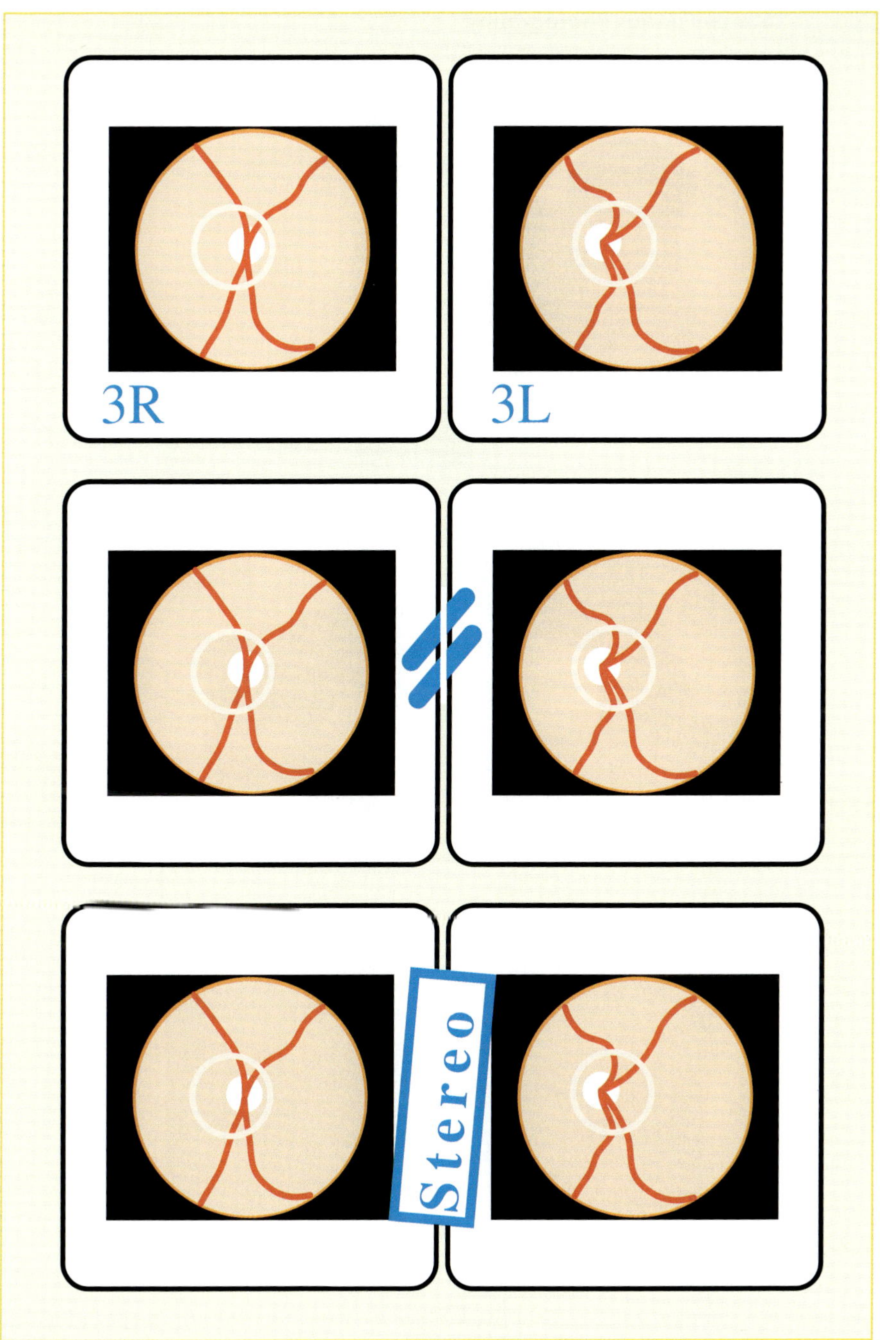

Figure 6–6 ○ Labeling conventions for indicating stereo on the pairs of 2 × 2 slides. Slide pairs labeled with sequential pair numbers and "L" and "R" (*top*), a simple set of lines (*middle*), or a rubber stamp with the word "stereo" (*bottom*).

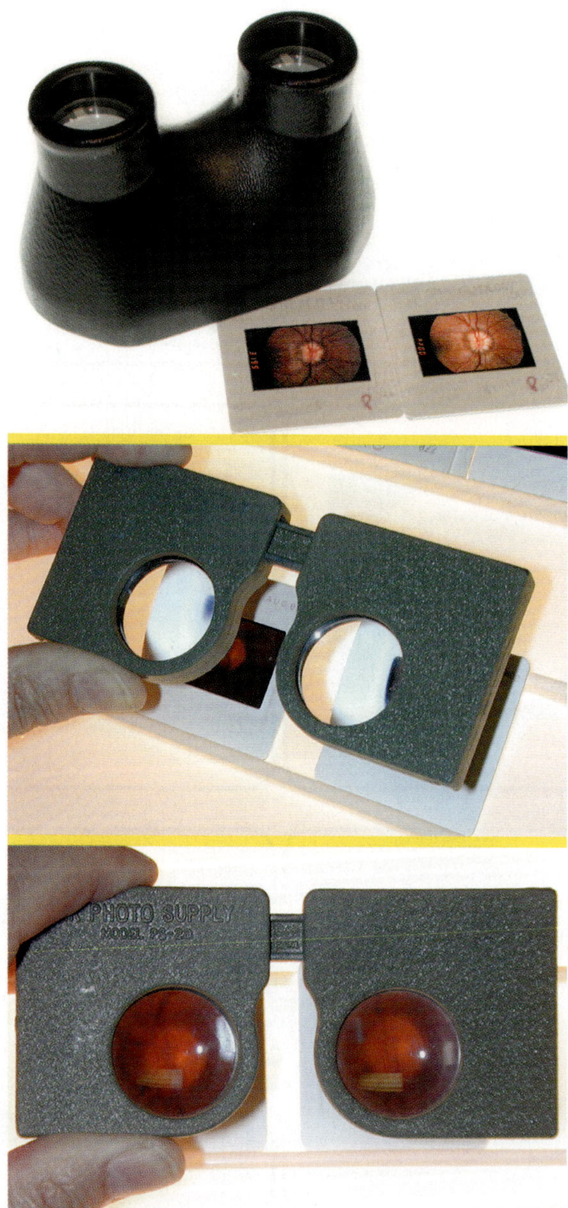

Figure 6–7 ○ Standard 2 × 2 stereo viewers allow you to lay two 35-mm slides side-by-side on a light table to view them in stereo (*top*). The best viewers have high-quality, two-element glass lenses; a comfortable interpupillary distance; and ample space for your nose (*center, bottom*). The Air Photo Supply Model PS-2a stereo viewer has variable interpupillary distance.

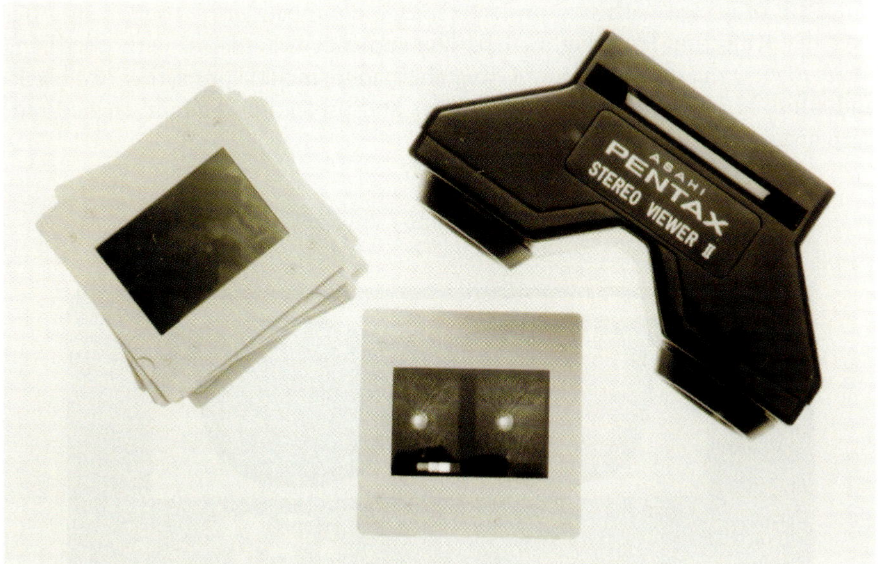

Figure 6–8 ○ A split-frame stereo viewer.

systems produce slides with the left image on the left, but a few systems produce slides with the image that is to be viewed with the left eye placed on the right side of the slide. Consequently, there are two types of split-frame stereo viewers. If you get a viewer with the wrong configuration of optics for the slides you are producing, you will get stereoscopically reversed image (e.g., disc cupping will be presented as an elevation).

Printing monochromatic stereo images as a single anaglyph image lets most viewers perceive the stereo image using red-cyan glasses (Fig. 6–9). The left image is printed in red, and the right in cyan. Anaglyph stereo allows images to be printed large, presenting more information than small side-by-side images. They may appear to be a black-and-white image with poor printing registration— you will see red or cyan "ghosts" to the left or right of the main image. Computer programs can be used to create red-cyan images. This technique is useful for the printed page, computer screens, computer projection, and slides. Anaglyphs were prepared on the computer for the *Stereo Atlas of Fluorescein and Indocyanine Green Angiography.*[6]

The key principle of stereo projection is the same as that of other stereo viewing strategies. As with all stereo viewing systems, each eye must be presented with an individual image. Stereo projection in ophthalmology can be performed with two polarized images projected onto a single lenticular screen. Two 2 × 2 slides are projected with two projectors, each equipped with a polarizing filter over the projection lens (Fig. 6–10). The audience uses glasses with polarizing filters to view the stereo images.[2] Other alternatives include projecting two black-and-white images through red-cyan filters and projecting digitally created red-cyan anaglyphs.

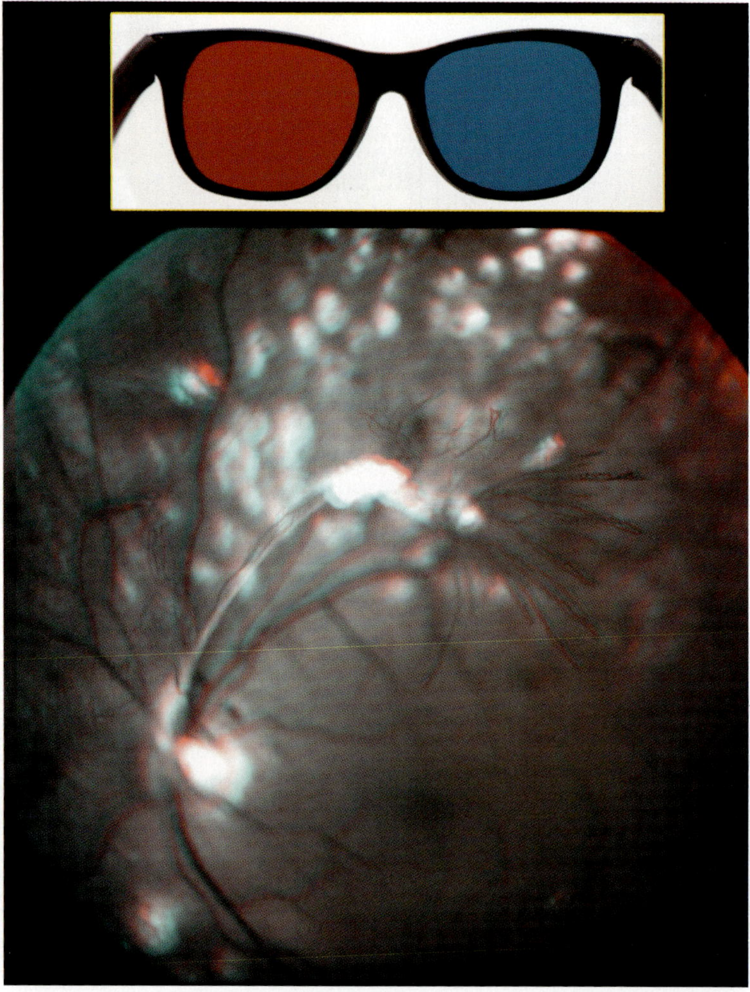

Figure 6–9 ○ Red-cyan glasses (*top*) are used to view a stereo anaglyph photograph of disc neovascularization from diabetic retinopathy (*bottom*).

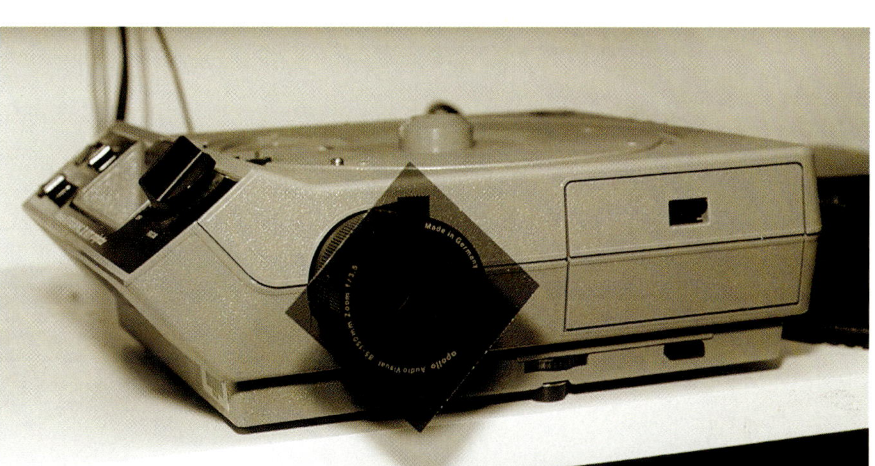

Figure 6–10 ○ One of the two 35-mm projectors with polarizing filters used for stereo projection.

The dynamic range and color saturation are very good on computer screens. Stereo images can be displayed on the monitor or printed on paper (from the computer image file), the same as for the standard viewing systems. Computers can be used to present stereo images either on a monitor or to a larger audience via a liquid crystal device (LCD) computer projector. Some type of stereo glasses are required for each system. All of the imaging systems for viewing small images will work with images displayed on computer monitors. Use viewing aids the same as you would for stereo images that are printed on paper or film transparency material. Side-by-side (small), side-by-side (larger than 60 mm), and anaglyph images are useful viewing methods. Although you can free-view small images, the granularity of the screen limits fine detail. However, monitor resolution is a limitation, as it is less than one-tenth that of 35-mm slide pairs. Zooming the image on the monitor may help to overcome the limits of screen resolution. Larger side-by-side images viewed with a four-mirror stereoscope provide good detail (Fig. 6–11).

Anaglyph images can easily be projected via computer projector or standard 35-mm projector onto any type of projection screen. Color fundus images may be computer projected and viewed through LCD glasses. This is currently the best way to see projected color fundus stereo images. Multiple viewers may experience the stereo affect at the same time using lenticular monitors. Lenticular monitors use a special screen and software to break the image into left and right views.

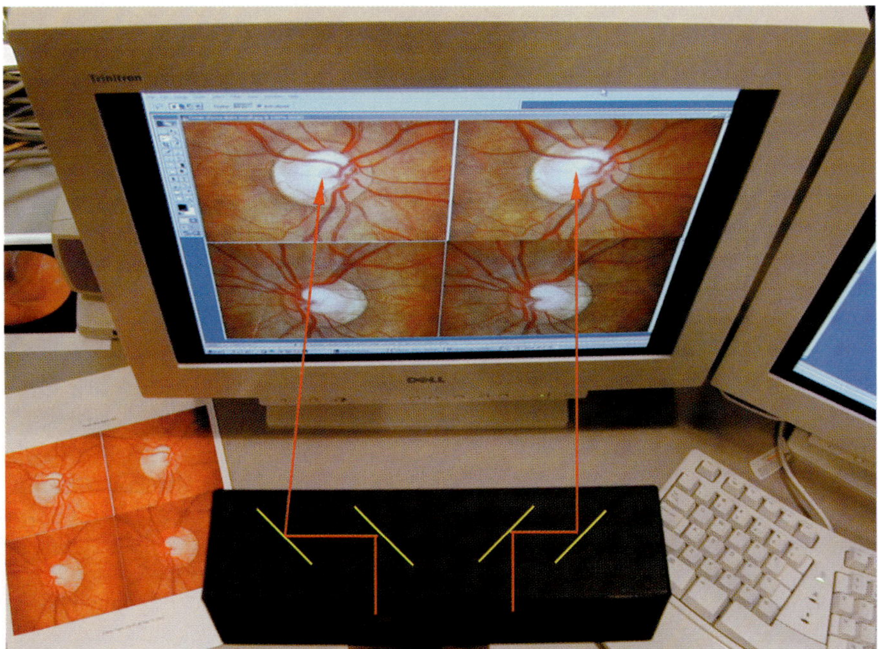

Figure 6–11 ○ A Brewster stereoscope. Note that one of the outer mirrors has an adjustable angle to permit viewing images of slightly different sizes.

Future Stereo Imaging in Ophthalmology

The value of the two images that make up a stereo pair is truly greater than the sum of the parts. The additional information that stereo imaging gives the clinician should not be underestimated.

The use of stereo images in telemedicine increases the diagnostic capabilities of the consulting physician. In the changing medical community, the ability to obtain multilevel and high-level consults without the patient needing to see each and every consultant physically will play an important role in the future of ophthalmic photography. With computer network capabilities, the ability to access a stereo view of the fundus of a patient in a remote location may become an accepted practice.

Simultaneous stereo camera images taken with reproducible stereo techniques permit high-quality image computer analysis of these images. Through disc analysis, the diagnosis of glaucoma may become possible even before functional field loss manifests itself. Thus the ability to photograph stereo images is a crucial skill. The ophthalmic photographer must have complete understanding and control of the theories and practices of ophthalmic stereo photography to ensure the ultimate care for the patient.

References

1. Allen L: Ocular fundus photography. Am J Ophthalmol 1964;57:13.
2. Saine PJ, Tyler ME: Ophthalmic Photography: Retinal Photography, Angiography and Electronic Imaging. Boston: Butterworth-Heinemann, 2002.
3. Walker BP: Photographic filing systems. Int Ophthalmol Clin 1976;16:2.
4. Ferwerda JG: The World of 3-D: A Practical Guide to Stereo Photography. Borger, The Netherlands: 3-D Book Productions, 1987.
5. Merin L: Construction and use of stereo viewers. J Ophthalmol Photog 1981;4:39.
6. Stevens RA, Saine PJ, Tyler ME: Stereo Atlas of Fluorescein and Indocyanine Green Angiography. Boston: Butterworth-Heinemann, 1999.

Chapter 7

Fundus Photography: Descriptive Interpretation

Introduction

Examining your initial fundus photographs is a bit like reviewing travel snapshots taken in a foreign land. You remember having taken the trip (the photographs in front of you are proof that you were there), yet the images seem strangely different. On reviewing them, you will discover new shapes, colors, and details that you may have failed to notice at the moment of exposure. And the more you study the images, the more you'll see.

This chapter uses fundus images of common retinal characteristics to orient you to the new landscape you will be photographing. Our intention is a short introduction to the visual characteristics of the normal and diseased fundus; this chapter is not meant to be a comprehensive guide to retinal abnormalities. You can learn more about the retina by reviewing your clinical photographs with your referring physician, by studying a comprehensive fundus atlas, and by attending continuing education seminars in ophthalmic photography. A greater understanding of the eye in normal and diseased states will enhance your fundus photography results.

Landmarks in the normal fundus and its variations begin the chapter. Abnormal maculae and optic discs are described, as are vascular abnormalities and various types of hemorrhages. We conclude with a potpourri of retinal abnormalities and a look at fundus photographs after retinal surgery.

The Normal Fundus

The easiest fundus landmark for orientation is the optic disc (Fig. 7–1). This somewhat oval, pink structure is located about 15 degrees nasal to the central

* This chapter is reproduced, with permission, from Saine PJ, Tyler ME: Ophthalmic Photography: Retinal Photography, Angiography, and Electronic Imaging, 2nd Edition. Boston: Butterworth-Heinemann, 2002, pp. 359–368.

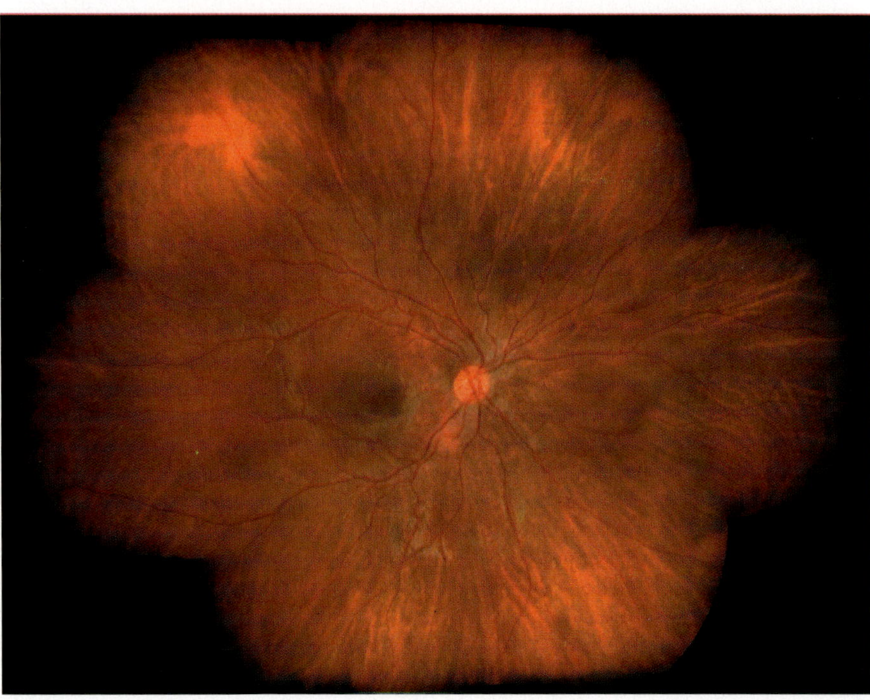

Figure 7–1 ○ Normal fundus, right eye. (FundusMap, a multi-image computer composite photoillustration, courtesy of Wake Forest University Eye Center and Richard E. Hackel, University of Michigan.)

visual axis (fovea). The optic disc overlies the scleral canal and is made up of a number of elements entering or leaving the eye:

1. *Blood vessels:* The central retinal artery emerges from the center of the disc and immediately divides to deliver blood to the four quadrants of the retina. The superior and inferior temporal branches (arcades) sweep around the fovea and roughly define the macula. The retinal veins form a similar pattern as they exit the eye at the optic disc. The optic disc can therefore always be found by tracing these vessels to their point of convergence.

2. *Axons:* The optic disc contains more than a million axons; these "wires" are cell processes that begin in the inner retina and converge to form the optic nerve, making a right-angle turn to exit the eye on their way to the brain. The fine capillaries that support these axons give the disc its pink color. These axons make up the neural rim of the optic disc, which in most individuals surrounds a central, whitish depression of variable size (the optic cup).

The visual axis of the eye intersects the retina at the fovea, the center of the macula. Photoreceptors are highly concentrated here to deliver the sharpest, clearest vision. The fovea is centered between the temporal vascular arcades and can be identified as a circular pigmented area slightly larger than the disc. The large number of axons extending radially from the center of the fovea cause a mound of increased retinal thickness, often identified by circular light reflexes on the smooth, innermost transparent retinal layer (the internal limiting membrane). To provide the clearest optical performance, axons from the temporal retina are carefully routed around the fovea. This strategy is the basis of the arc-shaped pattern of the nerve fiber layer. The axons can often be seen as fine striations sweeping toward the disc, especially above and below the disc, where the nerve fiber layer is thickest.

In lightly pigmented patients, the deeper choroidal circulation is evident. These vessels have a more random pattern and do not normally communicate with retinal vessels.

The Fundus: Normal Variations

The pigmentation (and thus the transparency) of the retinal pigment epithelium (RPE) may vary considerably among normal individuals, generally correlating with the degree of pigmentation elsewhere (e.g., skin, hair). Thus in the fundus of blond individuals, the choroidal vessels are easily seen (Fig. 7–2*A*). In darkly pigmented individuals, all choroidal details are hidden by the relatively opaque retinal pigment epithelium (Fig. 7–2*B*) In some subjects, there may be marked variations of pigmentation within the same fundus (Fig. 7–2*C*).

Congenital hypertrophy of the RPE (Fig. 7–2*D*) appears as characteristic grouped areas of darkly pigmented spots often described as *bear tracks*. This finding does not cause visual symptoms but is important because it must be distinguished from melanoma or other pigmented fundus lesions.

The optic nerve consists of over a million axons that begin in the retina, travel over the inner retina (as the nerve fiber layer), and exit the eye as the optic nerve. As the axons exit the eye, they acquire an insulating coating (myelin), which increases the speed and efficiency of data transfer. Occasionally, otherwise normal individuals will show aberrant myelinization of axons in the nerve fiber layer, producing feathery, superficial, white areas extending along the path of the nerve fiber layer (Fig. 7–2*E*).

In asteroid hyalosis, opaque white concretions (calcium soaps) are scattered throughout the vitreous. Despite their impressive appearance, they generally do not cause visual symptoms, although they can interfere with visualization of the retina (Fig. 7–2*F*).

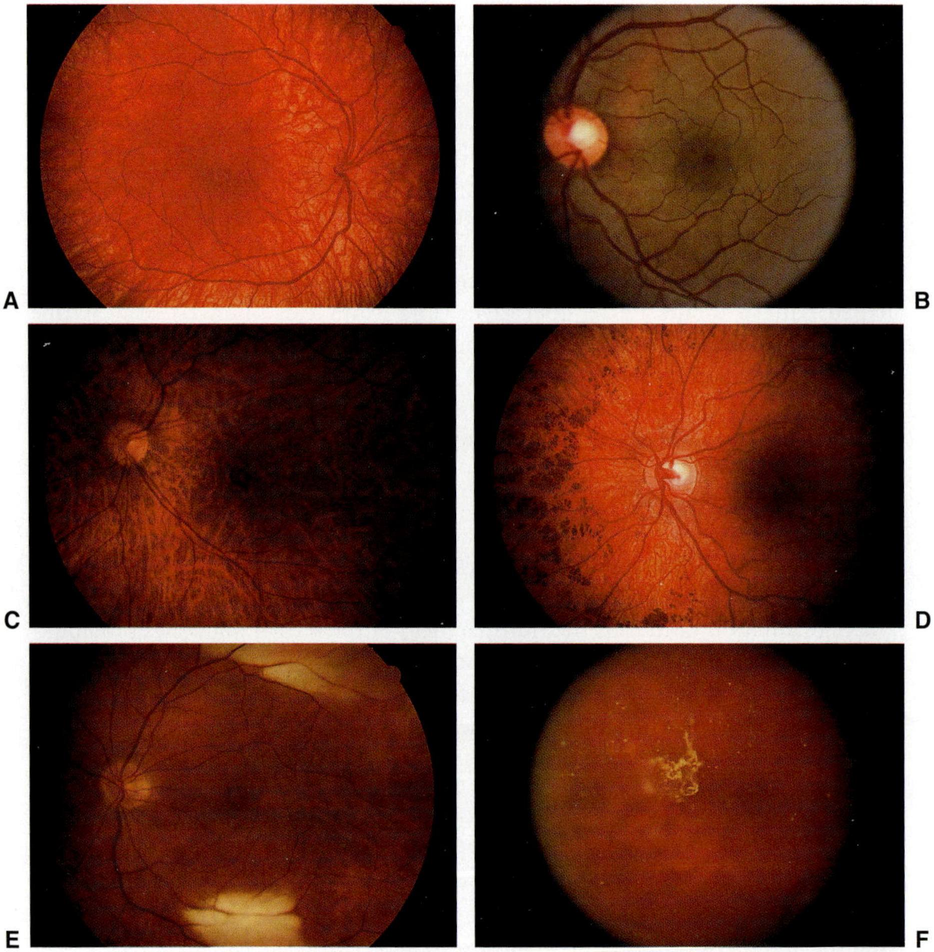

Figure 7–2 ○ Normal variations. *A,* Blond fundus, with transparent, lightly pigmented retinal pigment epithelium (RPE), showing the deep choroidal vessels. *B,* Highly pigmented RPE. *C,* Tigroid fundus shows variations in RPE. *D,* Congenital hypertrophy of the RPE. *E,* Myelinated nerve fiber layer. *F,* Asteroid hyalosis.

The Posterior Pole

In contrast to the water-tight retinal vessels, the vessels in the choriocapillaris are inherently leaky, though Bruch's membrane prevents this fluid from entering the subretinal space by providing the outer blood-retinal barrier. Bruch's membrane is a complex layer between the RPE and the choroid and is composed of elements from the base of the RPE and the choriocapillaris. A number of diseases damage

Bruch's membrane and the RPE. In age-related macular degeneration (ARMD), fluid may collect under the RPE, appearing as *soft drusen.* (Fig. 7–3*A*). Fluid also collects under the RPE in central serous retinopathy, a disease of young patients, and breaks through the RPE to collect under the neurosensory retina (Fig. 7–3*B*). Discontinuities in Bruch's membrane occur in many clinical entities, allowing choroidal vessels to grow into the sub-RPE and subretinal space (subretinal neovascular membrane). ARMD is a common cause of subretinal neovascularization and hemorrhage (Fig. 7–3*C*).

Myopic individuals of any age may also develop choroidal neovascular membranes. It is thought that in such large, myopic eyes, Bruch's membrane is stretched tenously thin (as suggested by the failure of the RPE to reach completely to the disc margin, resulting in a *myopic halo* around the disc) and is prone to breakage (Fig. 7–3*D*).

Many different diseases may cause the retinal vessels to become leaky, allowing blood components to seep into the deep retinal tissues. As the fluid portion resorbs, chalky-white hard exudates, or *edema residues,* are left behind. In the fovea, the dense radiating axons (Henle's nerve fiber layer) enclose the edema and create radial or wedge-shaped patterns. In other areas, rings of edema residue encircle the leaky spots (Fig. 7–3*E*). Diabetic retinopathy is a very common cause of these hard exudates.

Many ocular disorders may be associated with the growth of membranes at the innermost level (toward the center of the eye) of the retina. Contraction of these membranes results in macular pucker, or wrinkling, distorting vision (Fig. 7–3*F*).

The Optic Disc

In glaucoma, visual field defects result from axonal death. Axonal loss can be identified in the fundus as loss of the nerve fiber layer striations and enlargement of the central cup in the optic disc (Fig. 7–4*A*). In other forms of optic atrophy, the optic cup may change little but the normally pink neural rim becomes pale (Fig. 7–4*B*).

Acute disorders of the optic disc often result in swelling of the axons and supporting tissue, causing elevation of the disc and blurring of the disc margins (Fig. 7–4*C*). The cerebrospinal fluid that bathes the brain and spinal column also surrounds the optic nerve right up to the globe. Intracranial diseases can raise the pressure of this fluid and can cause bilateral disc swelling. Other common causes of disc swelling include anterior ischemic optic neuropathy and optic neuritis.

The optic disc may also be elevated by rock candy–like hyaline material buried in the axons of the optic disc. Visual field loss can occasionally result, but the finding is usually benign. In older individuals, this refractive material can

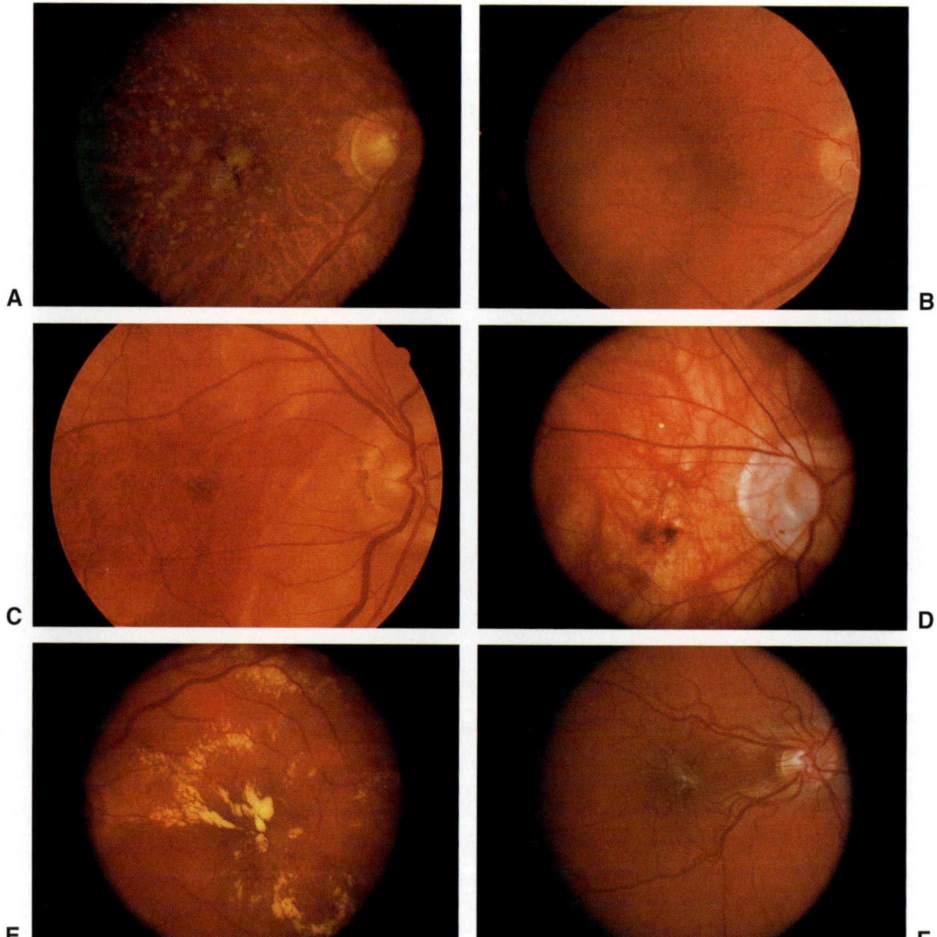

Figure 7–3 ○ The posterior pole. *A,* Age-related macular degeneration with soft drusen. *B,* Central serous chorioretinopathy. *C,* Subretinal neovascularization. *D,* Myopic halo or scleral crescent. *E,* Circinate retinopathy. *F,* Epiretinal membrane.

often be seen poking through the surface of the disc (Fig. 7–4*D*). In young patients, the material may be completely buried, and the disc elevation may be difficult to distinguish from true disc swelling (Fig. 7–4*E*).

Congenital malformations of the optic disc (such as an optic nerve coloboma) can result in bizarre appearances, with variable visual disfunction (Fig. 7–4*F*).

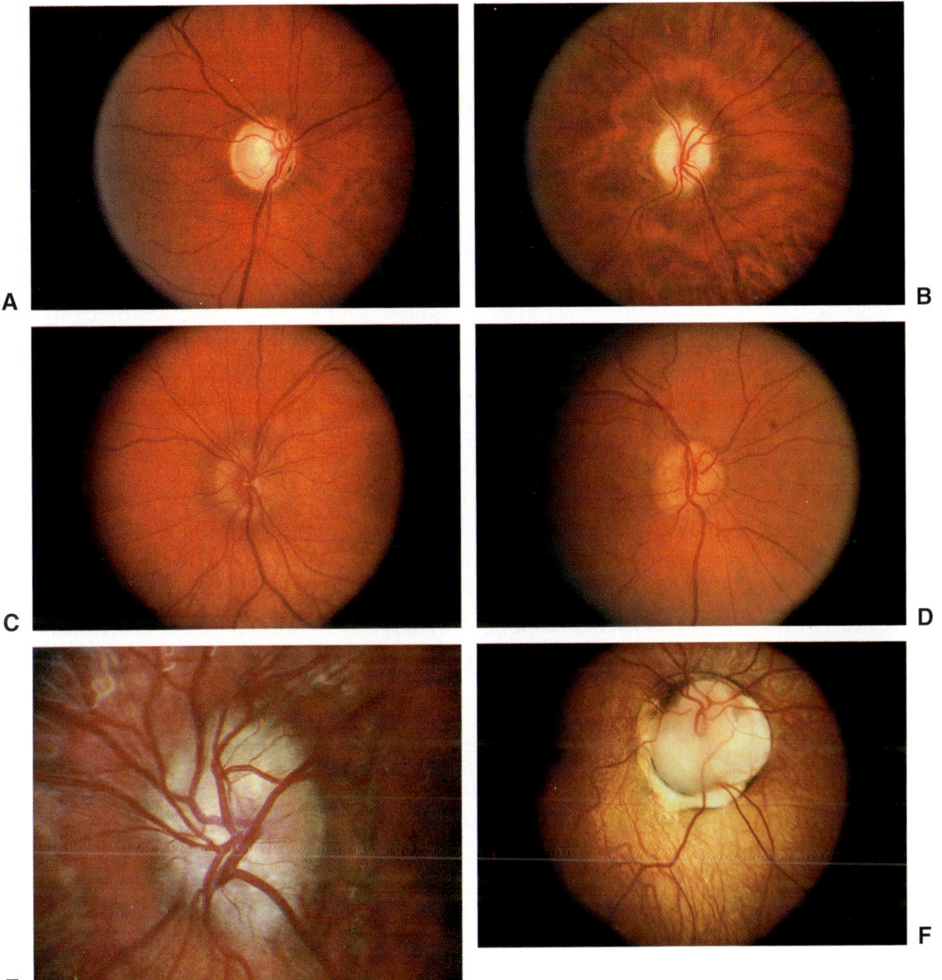

Figure 7–4 ○ The optic disc. *A,* Glaucomatous optic nerve. *B,* Optic atrophy. *C,* Optic disc edema. *D,* Drusen of the optic nerve. *E,* Buried drusen. *F,* Coloboma of the optic nerve.

Vascular Abnormalities

Infarction of the retina can occur if intravascular material (an embolus) lodges in the central retinal artery or its branches. Hollenhorst plaques are cholesterol crystals that commonly originate in the large carotid arteries in the neck and can be seen as glistening white, refractile material, often at arterial bifurcations (Fig. 7–5*A*). More proximal blockage of the central retinal artery can be identified acutely as an opaque, pale, macular swelling accentuating the choroidal red of the foveola, known as the *cherry red spot.* Following infarction, the normally transparent arterial wall may become opaque, appearing as a ghost vessel (Fig. 7–5*B*).

Retinal ischemia from vascular disorders such as diabetes may incite neovascularization. These new blood vessels grow into the vitreous from the disc (Fig. 7–5*C*) or elsewhere (Fig. 7–5*D*), resulting in vitreous hemorrhages and retinal traction detachments. A common early sign of ischemic diabetic retinopathy is segmental narrowing of retinal veins, creating venous beading. Figure 7–5*E* shows venous beading in a patient with radiation retinopathy.

Systemic hypertension causes stiffening and thickening of the retinal arterial walls, resulting in segmental narrowing as well as the appearance of venous discontinuity at artery-vein crossings (A-V nicking) (Fig. 7–5*F*).

Retinal Hemorrhages

Hemorrhages may occur at any retinal level. The shape of the hemorrhages is determined by the orientation and shape of the surrounding tissue structures at that level. Blood beneath the sensory retina (subretinal) can separate layers and spread out (Fig. 7–6*A*). Dot and blot hemorrhages are rounded by the deep structures in the retina (Fig. 7–6*B*). The orientation of the nerve fiber layer creates elongated flame-shaped hemorrhages (Fig. 7–6*C*). Blood on the surface of the retina (preretinal) obscures retinal details (Fig. 7–6*D*), its shape being determined by the apposition of the vitreous hyaloid face and the forces of gravity (Fig. 7–6*E*).

Figure 7–6*F* is a fundus photograph depicting the characteristic trauma-induced hemorrhages that occur in shaken baby syndrome.

Retinal Potpourri

Presumed ocular histoplasmosis syndrome presents with punched-out chorioretinal scars and peripapillary atrophy (Fig. 7–7*A*). Patients are generally asymptomatic unless they develop a third common finding: macular choroidal neovascualar membranes.

Ischemic retinal disorders may cause fluffy, superficial, white "cotton-wool" spots. These lesions are the result of swelling and opacification of the nerve fiber layer and may obscure the retinal details. Cotton-wool spots are likely areas of focal nerve fiber layer ischemia and are common in diabetic, hypertensive, and human immunodeficiency virus (HIV) retinopathy (Fig. 7–7*B*).

A common cause of blindness in HIV-infected patients is cytomegalovirus retinitis (Fig. 7–7*C*). Prompt treatment may prevent its progression to multiple retinal holes and retinal detachment.

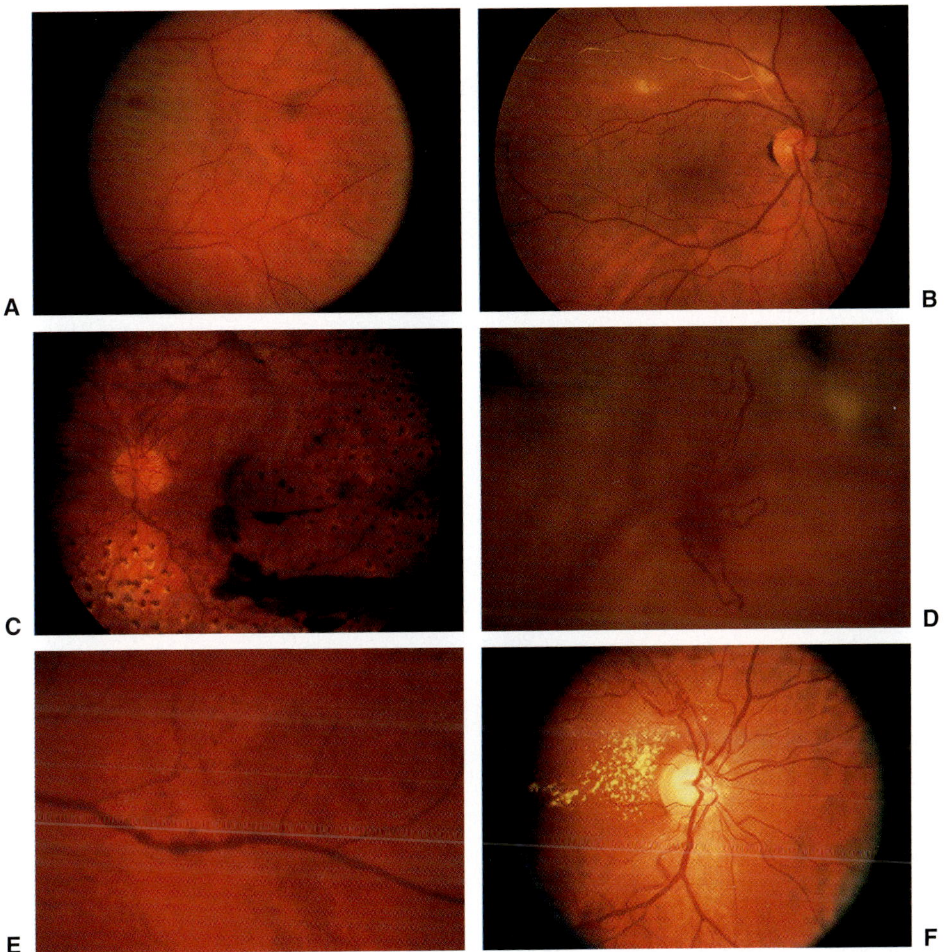

Figure 7–5 ○ Vascular abnormalities. *A,* Hollenhorst plaque. *B,* Central retinal artery occlusion. *C,* Neovascularization of the optic nerve. *D,* Neovascularization elsewhere. *E,* Venous beading. *F,* Arterial-venous crossing change.

Choroidal nevi (Fig. *7–7D*) are similar to moles on the skin. They are common and generally benign but must be distinguished from choroidal melanoma.

Angioid streaks are radial cracks in Bruch's membrane (Fig. *7–7E*). Because they are red and radiate from the disk, they may be mistaken for blood vessels (thus, "angioid"). Choroidal neovascular membranes may develop.

Retinitis pigmentosa represents a spectrum of retinal degenerative disorders often characterized by a peculiar "bony spicule" pigmentation of the peripheral retina (Fig. *7–7F*).

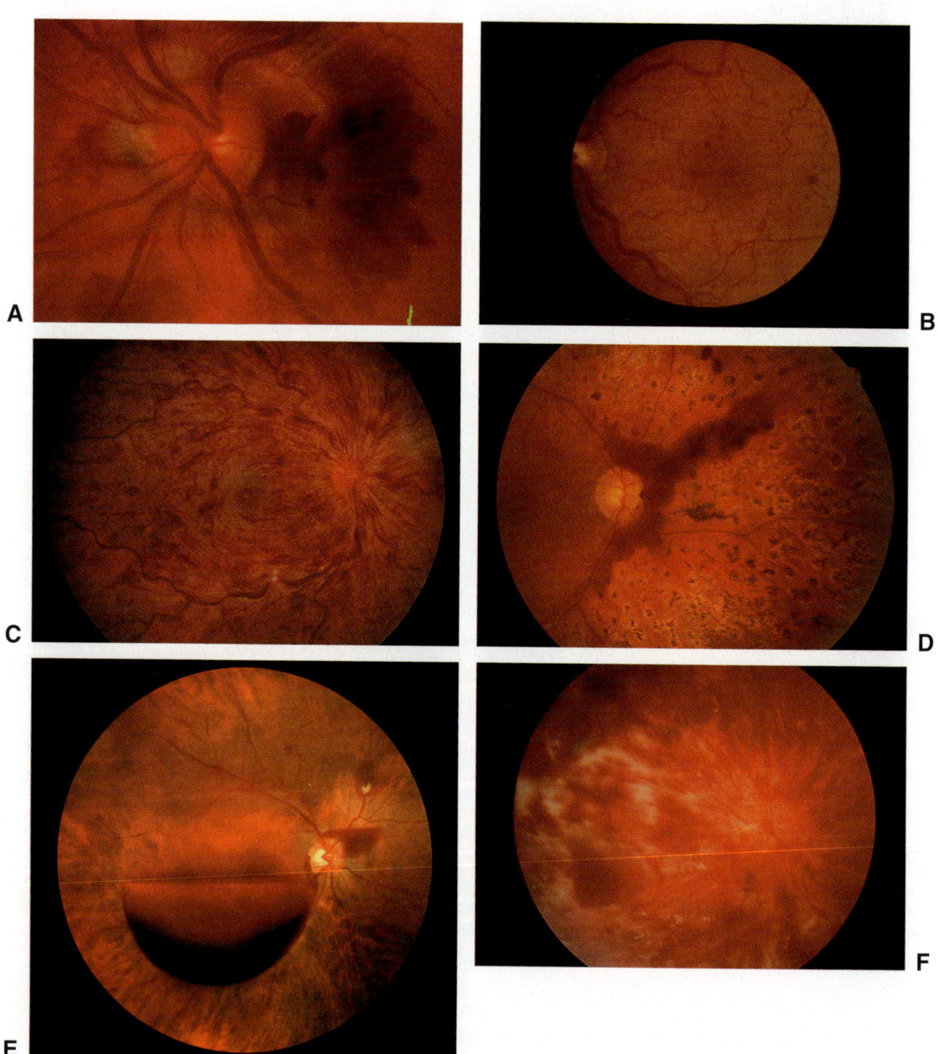

Figure 7–6 ○ Retinal hemorrhages. *A,* Subretinal blood. *B,* Dot and blot hemorrhages. *C,* Nerve fiber layer hemorrhages. *D,* Preretinal hemorrhage. *E,* Boat-shaped hemorrhage. *F,* Shaken baby syndrome. (Courtesy Wake Forest University Eye Center and Richard E. Hackel, University of Michigan.)

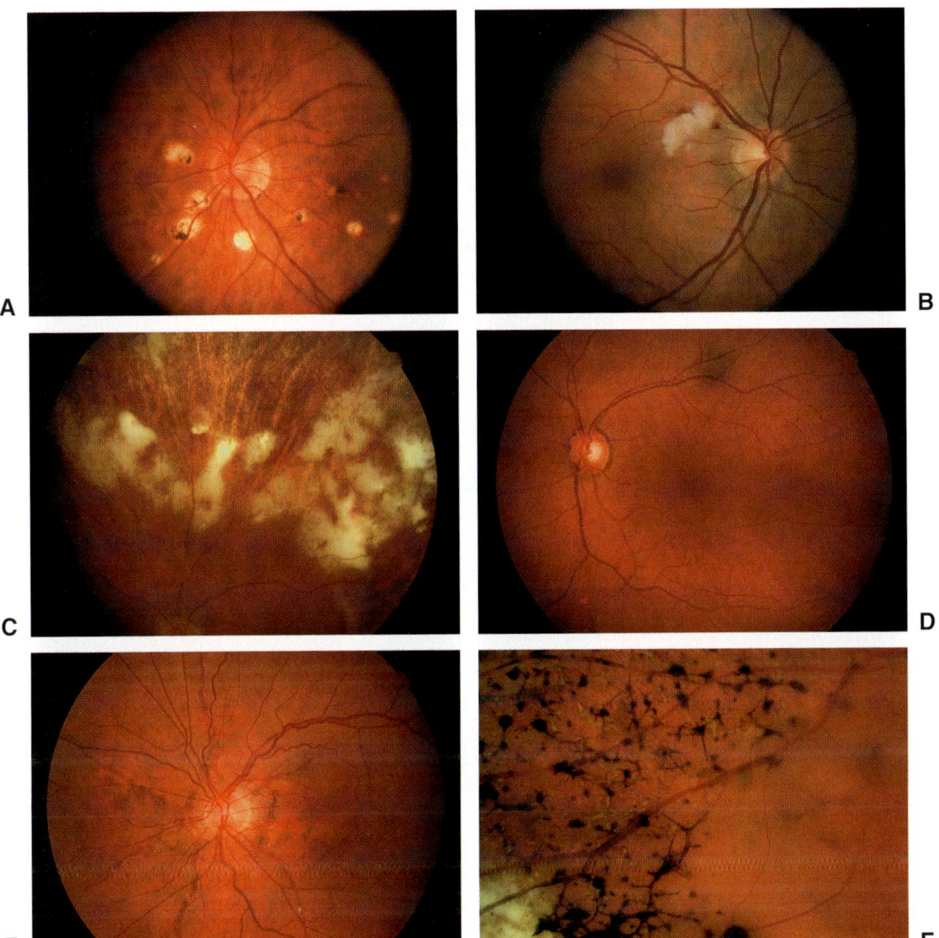

Figure 7–7 ○ Other retinal appearances. *A,* Presumed ocular histoplasmosis syndrome. *B,* Human immunodeficiency virus retinopathy. *C,* Cytomegalovirus retinitis. *D,* Retinal nevi. *E,* Angioid streaks. *F,* Retinitis pigmentosa.

The Surgical Fundus

Neovascularization in ischemic vascular disorders (especially diabetes) can frequently be prevented by selective destruction of ischemic retina with laser photocoagulation. Fresh laser spots appear as pale, soft white spots (Fig. 7–8*A*), with time developing into well-defined white areas with variable pigmentation (Fig. 7–8*B*).

Macular holes may develop if abnormal vitreous attachment and traction create a divot in the foveola. A cuff of retinal detachment is frequently seen (Fig. 7–8*C*).

Any break in the sensory retina may allow vitreous fluid to seep underneath, causing a retinal detachment (Fig. 7–8*D*). Surgery is required to close the break, often by using an external element to indent the globe beneath the break (Fig. 7–8*E*). In complicated cases, viscous silicone oil may be required to mechanically steamroller the retina back into position (Fig. 7–8*F*).

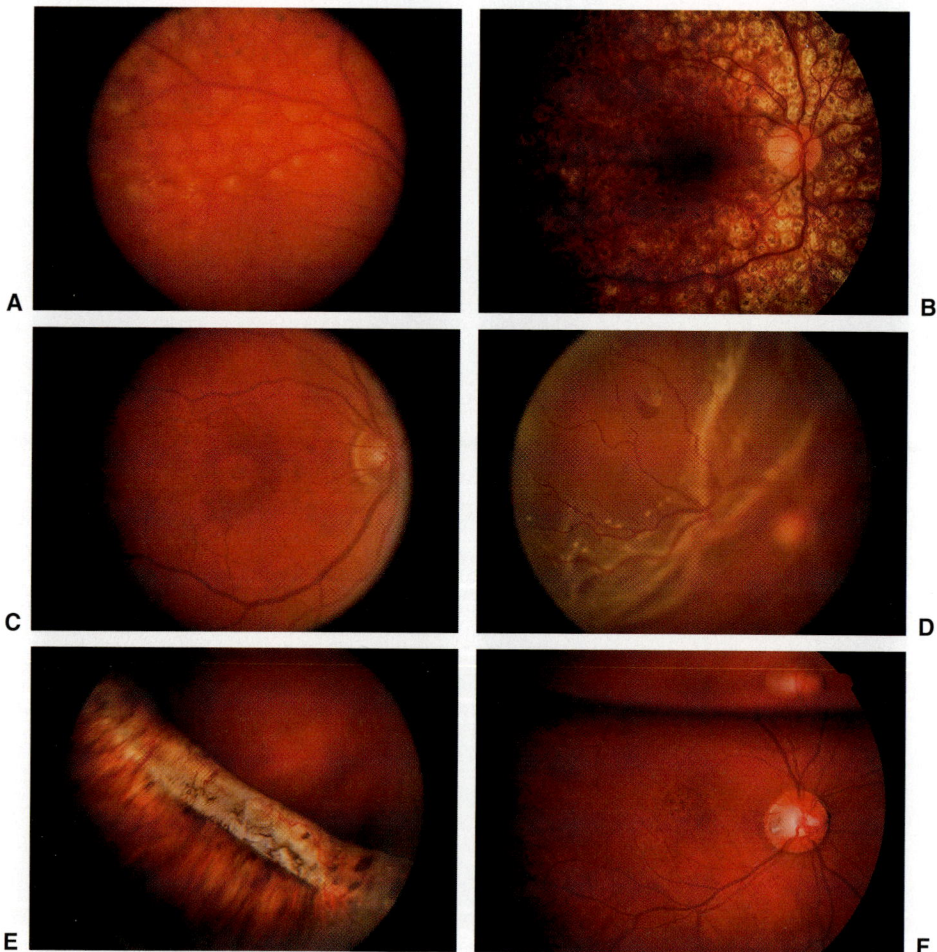

Figure 7–8 ○ The surgical fundus. *A,* Laser treatment. *B,* Laser treatment with time. *C,* Macular hole with operculum. *D,* Retinal detachment. *E,* Retinal appearance of a scleral buckle. *F,* Silicone oil vitreous replacement.

Ophthalmic photography integrates specialized photographic procedures with the clinical needs of the ophthalmologist. Successful ophthalmic photographers understand how and why their photographs are used.

Chapter 8

Digital Imaging Basics

The ophthalmic community was quick to embrace digital imaging for fluorescein angiography in the mid-1980s, but until recently, film has remained the medium of choice for color fundus photography in most practice settings. The rapid pace of improvement in electronic cameras, computer hardware, imaging software, and scanners has fueled the recent shift in preference toward digital imaging for fundus photography.

Digital imaging provides many advantages over traditional film-based photography. Computer technology offers a variety of powerful tools that can be used to enhance diagnostic information, share images across computer networks, and prepare them for academic presentation and publication. Digital fundus photographs can be enhanced in image-editing software to adjust brightness, contrast, color balance, and apparent sharpness. Computer measurement tools aid in the detection and quantification of pathologic features of the fundus. The computer monitor can display a retinal image that is larger and easier to see than the small frame of a 35-mm slide, enhancing patient education opportunities. Photographs can easily be e-mailed, displayed on web pages, imported into PowerPoint presentations, and printed on inkjet or dye-sublimation printers. Digital photographs can be printed within referral letters or reports and integrated in electronic medical records. Image files can be stored on computer hard drives, retrieved by image database programs, and archived to CD-R or other removable storage media. Digital technology has truly revolutionized the way in which we acquire and share fundus images (Fig. 8–1).

This chapter discusses the basics of digital imaging. Read this chapter if you are new to digital imaging or are seeking information on file size, file formats, or color management issues.

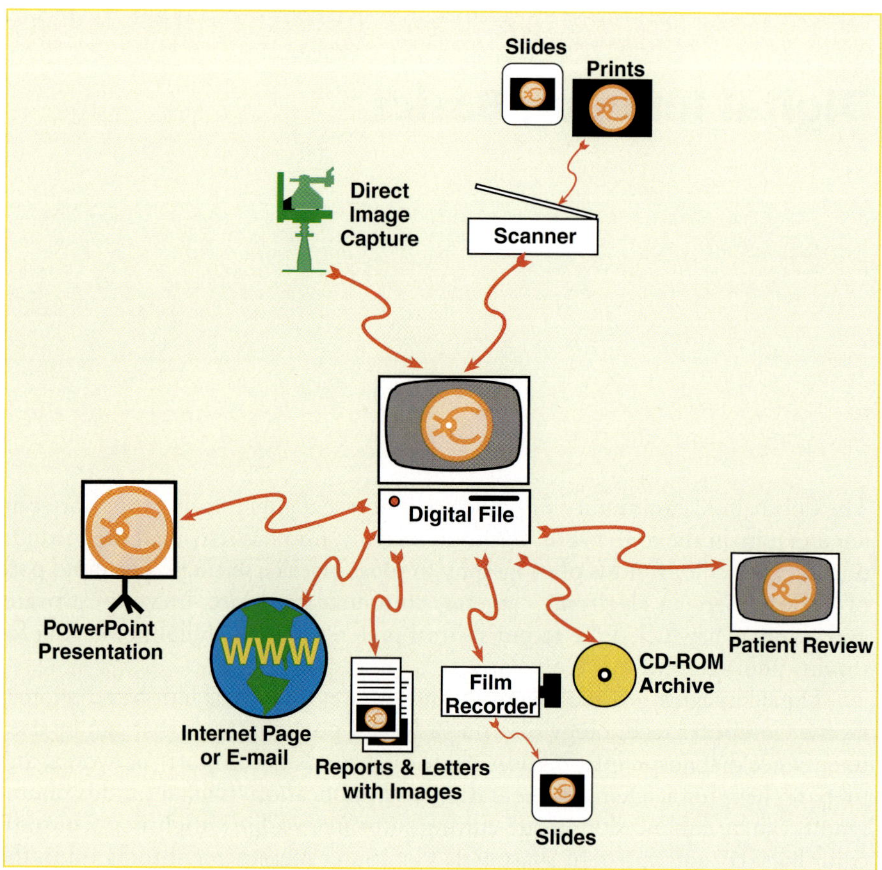

Figure 8–1 ○ There are a variety of ways to integrate digital-imaging techniques into your photographic workflow. Use digital cameras and scanners to digitize fundus photographs. Once an image is in electronic form, use computer software to enhance and prepare the image for a variety of output methods.

How Does Digital Imaging Work?

There are three major steps to the digital imaging process: image capture, image processing, and image output. Digital image capture describes the electronic recording of light information and its conversion to a set of numbers, which are then stored in an image file. Digital imaging is really just a new type of photography; as photographers, we still "write with light."

Digital images are captured by photosensitive imaging sensors in a camera or scanner (Fig. 8–2). The most common imaging array is a charge-coupled device, or CCD (see the accompanying box, "Image Sensors"). An *area CCD* is a square or rectangular matrix of photosensitive pixels arranged in rows and columns. Area CCDs are capable of capturing an entire image at once, which makes them suitable for flash photography or moving subjects. Area CCDs are used in still cameras such as the ones we use for fundus photography. *Linear CCDs* are thin rows of sensors that record a number of exposures as the array traverses or "scans" the subject. Linear CCDs are used in scanners.

Once an image has been captured and stored on a computer as numeric data, it can then be processed. Image processing uses computer software to manipulate the set of numbers that were created in the capture process to enhance the original image by adjusting contrast, exposure, color balance, cropping, and sharpness. Processing prepares the image for output. Image output involves converting the processed numeric data back into a viewable form for display, either onscreen or as printed hard copy. Screen output can take many forms, including computer monitor, remote display, e-mail, LCD projection, and web page display.

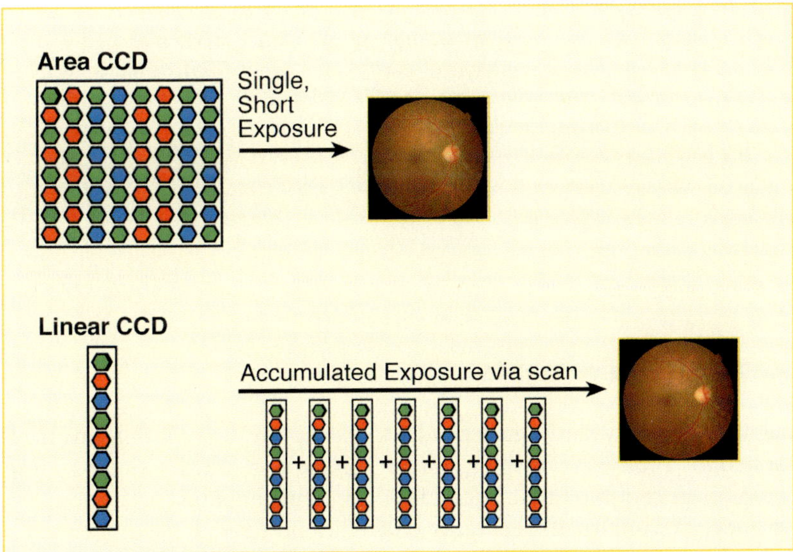

Figure 8–2 Two different types of CCD (charge-coupled device) imaging chips are used to acquire digital fundus photographs. An area CCD consists of rectangular grid of image sensors that captures an image in a single, short exposure. Area CCDs are used in digital cameras for direct capture of fundus photographs. Linear CCDs use a thin row of image sensors to construct an image sequentially, capturing many exposures as the imaging array moves across the subject. Linear CCDs are used in scanners.

Image Sensors

Since the 1970s, charge-coupled devices (CCD) have been used as image sensors in video and digital cameras. More recently, complementary metal oxide semiconductor (CMOS) sensors or "chips" have achieved improvements in image quality that rival CCDs. Both image sensor types are constructed of an array of photodetectors arranged in a grid or mosaic pattern of pixels. Each detector can capture only one color: red, green, or blue.

CCD and CMOS image sensor technologies each have advantages and disadvantages. CCDs are noted for their superior image quality. They exhibit greater light sensitivity, greater dynamic range, and less noise than CMOS chips but are more expensive to produce. There are only a handful of specialized fabrication facilities that are capable of producing CCDs.

CMOS chips are less expensive because they can be built by using common manufacturing techniques in high-volume facilities. CMOS chip architecture can include on-board analog-to-digital conversion and image processing, while the typical CCD device requires multiple support chips to provide the same functionality. CMOS image sensors use less energy and are not as susceptible to blooming and smearing of bright highlights. Despite these advantages, their poor low-light sensitivity and noisier image quality have relegated them to use in low-end image capture systems, but that is beginning to change.

A revolutionary new type of image sensor, dubbed the Foveon X3, was introduced in 2002. This chip design uses three separate photodetector layers arranged in a stack and captures full color information at each pixel location. This architecture may be capable of delivering sharper images than CCD or CMOS sensors with the same number of pixels. This emerging technology is promising.

The battle between these image sensor technologies is likely to continue. Both CCD and CMOS technologies continue to improve at a rapid pace, and it is likely that we will see continued improvements in the cameras and scanners we use for fundus imaging.

Hardware Requirements

Digital imaging is very hardware dependent. The capture device is only one hardware component of a complete imaging system. A basic system will require a computer and monitor. A computer that is used for digital imaging must have enough speed and memory to complete the necessary tasks efficiently. Peripheral input and output devices, such as cameras, scanners, and printers, can be added to expand the imaging capabilities of the basic system. When choosing a computer for imaging purposes, RAM, hard disk capacity, and auxiliary storage devices are important considerations because high-resolution image files can be quite large and may consume significant system resources. All components of a digital system need to be compatible with one another.

- **Computer.** Today's entry-level computers are designed to handle digital music, video, and pictures and are shipping with at least 256 megabytes (MB) of RAM, a 40- to 80-gigabyte (GB) hard drive, and a CD-R/RW drive for auxiliary storage. This is enough power and storage for many imaging needs. Midrange and high-end computers supply appropriate computing power, speed, and storage.
- **RAM.** Efficient processing of digital images may require a considerable amount of RAM (Fig. 8–3). A computer with 64 MB of RAM may be enough to handle small files intended for screen display or web use but would struggle with large image files. Large images require significant amounts of memory, so we recommend using a computer that has 3–5 times the maximum image file size in memory available for processing. Today's best CCD capture devices are capable of 3k by 2k (and higher) resolution. An image file this size is roughly 18 MB. For professional imaging use, it pays to get a powerful computer with at least 512 MB of RAM. High-end image-editing programs require enough RAM to hold multiple copies of the image for processing in layers or to undo changes. Plan accordingly to ensure that you have enough memory for your imaging needs.
- **Monitor.** A high-quality monitor that is capable of displaying 24-bit color is necessary for viewing and editing images. A video card with additional memory is useful for allowing the monitor to do its job efficiently without sharing RAM with the computer—RAM that could be better used for image processing. Calibrating the display so that it comes as close as possible to the color output of a printing device allows the most accurate color reproduction. Monitors that support XGA resolution (Table 8–1) or higher are appropriate for viewing and editing digital images.
- **Hard Drive.** A large-capacity hard drive or a second drive dedicated to image files will provide enough storage for high-volume use.
- **Storage.** An auxiliary storage drive is essential for archiving or transporting image files. Today's storage standard is the CD-R/RW drive, which is capable of handling 700 MB of storage per disk. The CD format is also useful for exporting and distributing photo files, since almost all computers are capable of reading CDs. DVD-RW is a newer alternative that offers greater storage capacity than CD. Double-sided DVD disks currently have a capacity of up to 9.4 GB.
- **Operating System.** Apple's Macintosh platform has traditionally excelled in high-end graphics and digital imaging use, but both Mac and Microsoft Windows operating systems (OS) can handle most fundus imaging needs. Check to see whether the applications you wish to use will run on your operating system. Another important consideration is to make sure that the OS is up-to-date and compatible with the current peripheral connection technology and drivers. Drivers are files that enable the computer and peripheral devices to communicate with one another.

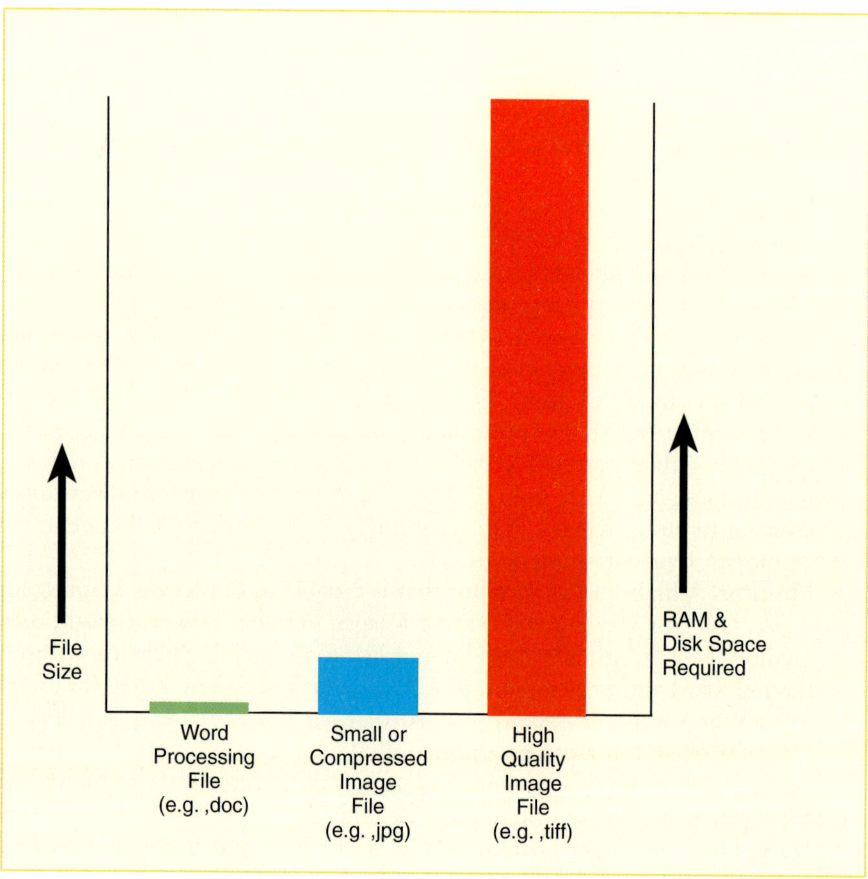

Figure 8–3 ◯ High-quality digital image files are typically much larger than word-processing or other common document types and place a greater burden on computer system resources. As file size increases, more RAM (random access memory) and more hard drive space are necessary for image editing and file storage.

Table 8–1
Monitor Resolution Standards

VGA	640 × 480
SVGA	800 × 600
XGA	1024 × 768
SXGA	1280 × 1024
UXGA	1600 × 1200

- **Connectivity.** A computer needs to have the appropriate data port connectors to attach all necessary capture and output devices. USB, SCSI, and FireWire ports may be necessary depending on the peripheral hardware being used. New, faster connection standards are being developed to improve performance.

Resolution

Managing resolution is a fundamental part of the digital imaging process. Concepts of resolution and the terminology used to describe it can lead to some confusion. In the most basic sense, resolution relates to the amount of detail contained in an image. In digital imaging, resolution refers to the number of specific points of picture information contained in an image file. These points are known as picture elements, or *pixels* (Fig. 8–4). The number of pixels in an image, or pixel

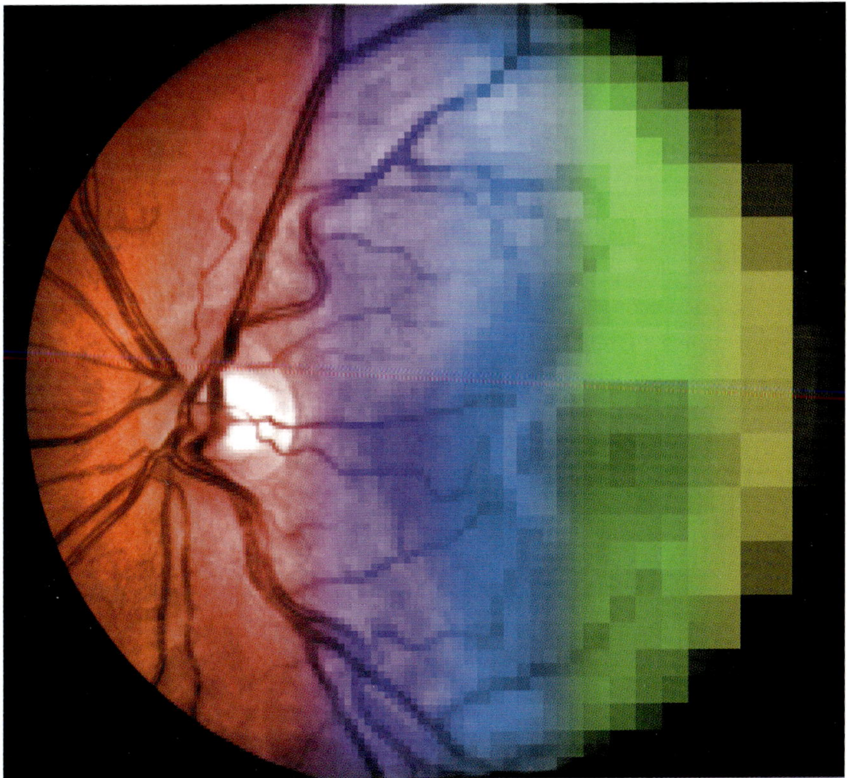

Figure 8–4 ○ Digital photographs are made up of individual picture elements or pixels. Image resolution directly relates to the number of pixels contained in an image. As pixel count decreases, detail is lost and individual pixels become more prominent.

count, has an effect on both resolution and file size. High-resolution images contain a relatively high number of pixels and can exhibit great image detail. When an image is low in resolution or has too few pixels for a given use, the pixels will be large and quite visible as small blocks or "jaggies." A high-resolution image would have to be magnified before individual pixels would become noticeable. Because pixel count also affects file size, image resolution should be matched to output requirements to maintain efficiency in image processing and file storage.

Bit depth, which is sometimes referred to as brightness resolution, also has an effect on the perceived quality of an image. A *bit*, or binary digit, is the smallest unit of digital information. Bit depth refers to the number of bits or brightness levels that are recorded for each pixel in an image file. A 1-bit value (2^1) for a gray-scale image would consist of two brightness levels: 0 (pure black) and 1 (pure white). An 8-bit (2^8) image can contain up to 256 brightness levels. Gray-scale images are typically 8-bit and can display 256 shades of gray (Fig. 8–5). Most modern color input devices will capture 8 bits for each of the primary color channels: red, green, and blue. The result is commonly referred to as *24-bit color* and results in over 16 million color possibilities (Fig. 8–6). Photographic images should be captured and displayed in at least 24-bit color. The latest generation of digital cameras and scanners are capable of capturing at higher bit depth numbers of 10, 12, or 14 bits per color (30-bit, 36-bit, and 42-bit color). Although most current monitors and printers are limited to 24-bit color output, capture at higher bit depth results in extra data that can reduce noise, improve exposure latitude, and increase detail in shadows and highlights.

One of the reasons why resolution might seem confusing is that it can be expressed in different ways. *Pixel dimensions* refer to the number of pixels in an image. An image that is 1600 pixels wide by 1200 pixels high would have pixel dimensions of 1600 × 1200. Resolution is also expressed in *pixels per inch (ppi)*. If your intended output is a print, then ppi is useful for determining the resolution and physical dimensions of the printed image. For example, the same image with a pixel dimension of 1600 × 1200 would print at a physical size of 8 × 6 inches with the resolution set at 200 ppi.

Screen resolution is quite different from print resolution. As output devices, monitors do not recognize the number of pixels per inch, only the pixel dimensions of an image. Monitor resolution varies and is user-adjustable for pixel dimensions and bit depth. Because of these variables, images with the same resolution will appear different in size on monitors with different sizes or resolution settings. When capturing or preparing an image for screen display, pixel dimensions are a more appropriate measure of resolution.

Some hardware manufacturers and imaging professionals also use the term *dots per inch (dpi)* to refer to image resolution. They often mean the same thing as pixels per inch, but this can be confusing because dpi is also used to describe

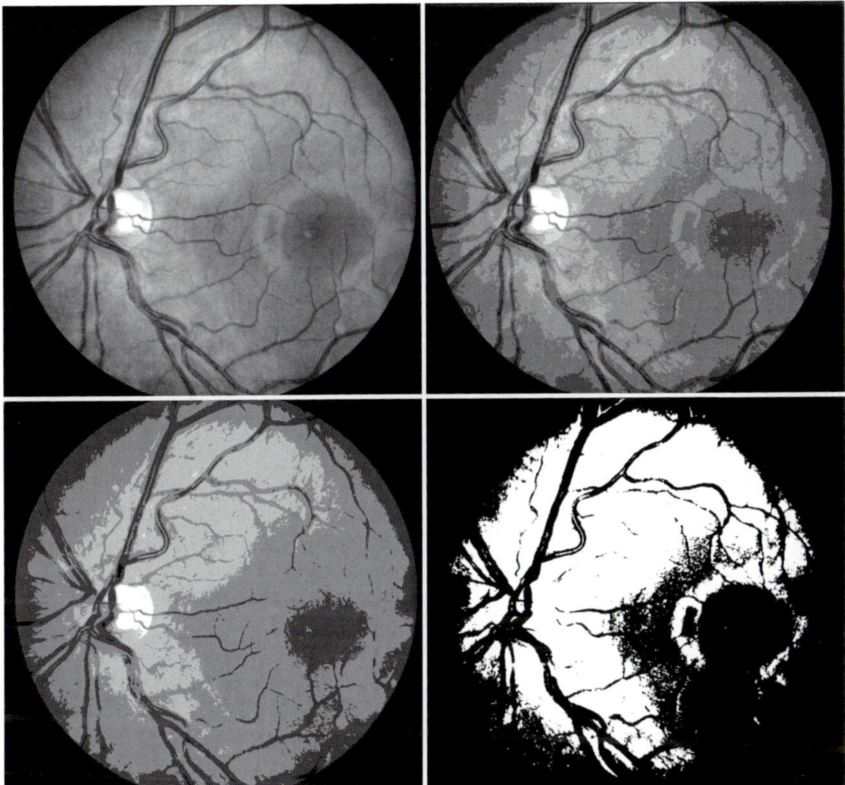

Figure 8–5 ○ Gray-scale bit-depth. *Top left*, 8-bit image displays 256 brightness levels. *Top right*, 3-bit image, eight brightness levels. *Bottom left*, 2-bit image, four brightness levels. *Bottom right*, 1-bit image, two brightness levels.

printer resolution. In some cases, printer dpi is a completely different number and should not be confused with image ppi.

Resizing: Scaling Versus Resampling

When describing resolution, we also need to consider sizing. Scaling or resampling an image is often necessary to size it properly for a given display or output resolution. A digital image file does not really have a physical size until you map the pixels to an output device. *Scaling* is the best way to resize an image while maintaining quality. Scaling does not affect the pixel count of the image. It simply stretches or compresses the pixels to fill a particular physical dimension. The size of the pixels

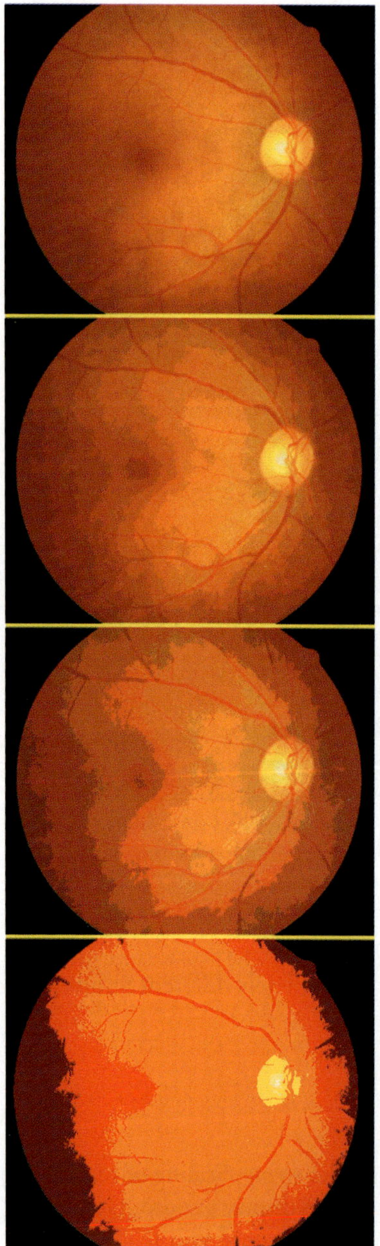

Figure 8–6 ○ Color bit depth. *Top*, 24-bit color displays over 16 million color possibilities. *Second*, 8-bit, 256 colors. *Third*, 4-bit, 16 colors. *Bottom*, 2-bit, 4 colors. Fundus images reproduce well at 24-bit (or greater) color.

themselves will increase or decrease accordingly. Dragging the corner sizing handles to increase or decrease image size in a page layout or presentation program is a common method of scaling. In this case, you are scaling an image by how it looks within a page layout.

You can also scale an image by specifying the size in inches or centimeters for printing. If you have an image with a pixel count of 1200 × 900, resizing would allow you to specify the physical dimensions for printing. Sizing this image for printing at a size of 4 × 3 inches would result in a resolution of 300 ppi. Increasing the print size to 8 × 6 inches would reduce the resolution to 150 ppi. If you need an image printed at this physical size with a higher resolution, you have two choices: reacquire the image at a higher resolution or resample it. Scaling can be specified at capture when scanning.

Resampling is another way to resize an image (Fig. 8–7). Unlike scaling, resampling changes the total number of pixels to either increase or decrease the resolution in ppi. Downsampling to resize an image is acceptable; it simply means discarding pixels to reach the desired resolution. This is commonly performed on high-resolution images that are being prepared for internet use. High-resolution images require long download times and are unnecessary for screen display. Images with pixel dimensions greater than the resolution of the monitor will yield no additional image quality.

Upsampling, or increasing the number of pixels through interpolation, will not create new detail. Upsampling asks the software program to invent pixels that do not exist. Although image-editing programs use sophisticated algorithms to upsample in this manner, the results may be disappointing. Resampling might not actually give you the expected increase in resolution. Yes, the pixel count will be higher, but detail will not increase. When you need to resample, try to keep the amount of upsampling to a minimum.

Selecting the best resolution for a given use is often a compromise. Interpolation or resampling is lurking everywhere. Scanners interpolate unless the scan resolution is set at the (full) optical resolution of the scanner. Scanning at a setting that is higher or lower than optical resolution will result in pixels being discarded or manufactured by the driver software. Inkjet printers also interpolate image data to determine a drop pattern for blending colors. Some interpolation in digital imaging may be unavoidable. For best results, however, try to limit the number of times that interpolation is performed throughout the imaging chain.

File Formats

Once you have acquired images, you might need to save or convert them to an appropriate file format for editing or output. Many imaging applications will save images in a native file format that is specific to that particular program.

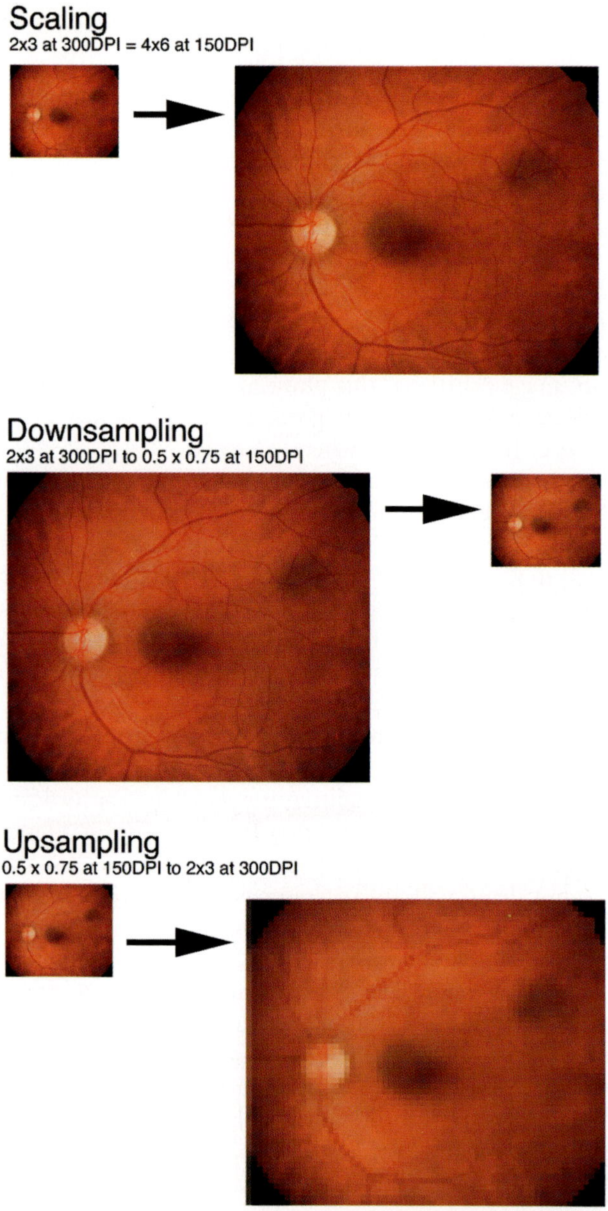

Scaling
2x3 at 300DPI = 4x6 at 150DPI

Downsampling
2x3 at 300DPI to 0.5 x 0.75 at 150DPI

Upsampling
0.5 x 0.75 at 150DPI to 2x3 at 300DPI

Figure 8–7 ○ There are various methods of resizing an image for output. Scaling simply defines a linear dimension, and the pixels expand or contract to fill the specified space. An image with pixel dimensions of 600×900 can be printed 2×3 inches in size at 300 dpi. The same image can be scaled for a different print size of 4×6 inches, at 150 dpi. The total number of pixels has not changed, but they are stretched to fit the new print dimensions. Downsampling is often used to reduce image size for a specific output resolution. It works by discarding pixels to achieve the desired size. Downsampling reduced our 2×3 inch, 300 dpi image to a new size of 0.5×0.75 inches at 150 dpi (75×112 pixels). Image quality at this size is still acceptable, even though the pixel count is much lower. Upsampling usually results in quality loss. Notice the decreased amount of fine detail and the visible pixels (jaggies) that result from upsampling.

These file formats are not always readable by other software applications, especially across platforms (from Macintosh to Windows and vice versa). In scanning, editing, or exporting images for presentation, e-mail, or web use, it is important to choose a file format that is suited for the job at hand (Table 8–2).

The format you choose for saving an image will have a significant effect on file size. File size is an important consideration, especially in dealing with a large number of image files. Different file formats provide varying degrees of data compression, which can affect image quality. There are two types of data compression: lossless and lossy. *Lossless* compression can achieve about a 2:1 compression ratio, but the reconstructed image is identical to the original. *Lossy* compression offers higher compression rates and smaller file sizes, but the loss of data is sometimes visible to the eye. The most commonly used universal file formats are TIFF and JPEG. TIFF (lossless) is a good choice for archiving important images. The JPEG (lossy) format is useful for compressing images (smaller file size) for transfer over the Internet.

Cross-Platform Formats

JPEG

JPEG (*.jpg) is one of the most commonly used image file formats. Almost all programs that handle images in both the PC and Macintosh environments are capable of opening and saving JPEG files. Developed by the Joint Photographic Experts Group, this file format uses a lossy compression technique that can significantly reduce image file sizes. JPEG compression can reduce a file to as much as 5% of its original file size. Too much compression, however, will significantly reduce image quality. The amount of compression is selectable in most

Table 8–2
Suggested File Formats

Image Use	Preferred Format	Acceptable Format
Archive master image	TIFF	PNG, PSD
www: continuous-tone photos	JPEG	GIF (gray scale)
www: contains line art	GIF	
www: with transparent background	GIF	
E-mail	JPEG	GIF
Presentation graphics (PowerPoint, etc.)	JPEG	TIFF, PNG
Word processing	JPEG	BMP, TIFF
DTP (PageMaker, Publisher, Quark, etc.)	TIFF	EPS
PC-to-Macintosh transfer	TIFF	PICT, JPEG
Macintosh-to-PC transfer	TIFF	BMP, JPEG

imaging software programs, so the user can determine which is more important: compression or quality (Fig. 8–8). The JPEG format is particularly useful for images that are intended for Internet use. It works well on both full-color and gray-scale photographic images but is not recommended for text or line art.

Because JPEG relies on a lossy compression scheme, it is important to note that image quality can be lost *each* time an image is altered and then saved in this format (simply opening but not resaving a JPEG image does not have this effect). If you expect to edit and save changes frequently, it is better to use a lossless format while editing. Once editing is completed, a final save in the JPEG format will compress the file while keeping data loss to a minimum.

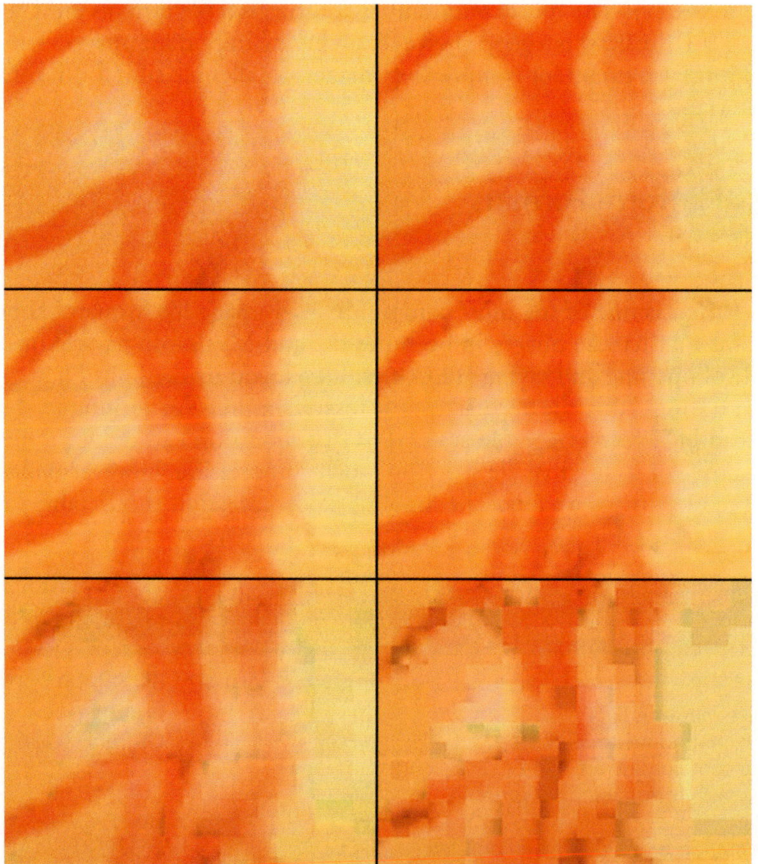

Figure 8–8 ○ JPEG compression comparison. *Top left,* The original lossless image. *Top right,* Quality setting: 9 on a scale of 10. *Center left,* Quality setting: 7. *Center right,* Quality setting: 5. *Bottom left,* Quality setting: 3. *Bottom right,* Quality setting: 1. Notice that image quality begins to degrade significantly at settings below 5.

TIFF

TIFF (*.tif), which stands for Tagged Image File Format, is a universal file format that is supported by many applications and computer platforms. It is useful for saving master copies of important images. It is a popular choice for working with images in an image-editing application. The major disadvantage to this format is that it results in a large file size. The TIFF format supports optional LZW compression, which is a lossless compression technique that nominally reduces file size while maintaining image quality. This compression technique does not compress file size enough for e-mail or web use. Furthermore, not all graphics programs recognize LZW compression and might not be able to open compressed TIFF files. Uncompressed TIFF files are popular for archiving and publication purposes.

GIF

GIF (*.gif), which stands for Graphics Interchange Format, was originally designed for Internet use. GIF also uses lossless LZW compression, but images are limited to 256 colors, which makes this format a poor choice for 24-bit color photographic images. The GIF format is best suited for simple graphics or gray-scale photographic images.

EPS

EPS (*.eps), which stands for Encapsulated PostScript, is a format that is used in high-end publishing and graphics production. The file contains a PostScript description that tells the printing device how to output the image. EPS files may contain an optional bitmap image to aid in page layout. Some programs will open and save in EPS format, but not all support saving the vector instructions for printing.

PNG

PNG (*.png), which stands for Portable Network Graphics, was designed as an alternative to the GIF format. It uses LZW compression as GIF does but is not limited to 256 colors. File sizes are larger than those of JPEG or GIF but smaller than those of TIFF with similar quality.

PDF

PDF (*.pdf), which stands for Portable Document Format, is the file format used by Adobe Acrobat Reader, a universal, cross-platform electronic document reader. PDF files can contain both vector and bitmap graphics (see the accompanying box, "Bitmap and Vector Image Formats").

> ### *Bitmap and Vector Image Formats*
>
> *Two main types of images are used in computer graphics: bitmap and vector. A basic understanding of these two image types will help if you want to combine fundus photographs with other graphical elements.*
>
> *Any image that we capture with a digital camera or scanner is a bitmap or raster image. Bitmap images are resolution-dependent, meaning that they are built by using a fixed number of pixels arranged in a grid pattern. Image-editing programs such as Photoshop use bitmap images to render photorealistic detail. Digital fundus photographs are bitmap images.*
>
> *Vector images are resolution-independent objects defined by mathematical formulas, as opposed to pixels. The formulas provide a set of instructions for drawing the image based on lines, curves, shape, color, fill, and location. They can be scaled and printed to any size without increasing file size or losing detail. Fonts are an example of vector objects. Vector objects are useful for rendering logos, clip art, text, arrows, and other geometric shapes. Vector data cannot reproduce photorealistic images.*
>
> *Metafile formats, produced by web browsers (e.g., Netscape and Internet Explorer), presentation software (e.g., PowerPoint), and desktop publishing programs (e.g., PageMaker and Quark XPress) can contain a combination of bitmap, vector data, and text, combining elements of each file type for final display.*

Platform-Specific Formats

These file formats are specific to their respective operating platforms. They are not intended as cross-platform formats, although most good imaging programs will be able to open files in either Windows or MacOS.

BMP

The Windows bitmap format (*.bmp) is the basic imaging format used in Window-based computers. It is a lossless format with large file sizes. It is most commonly used for images that will be displayed as Windows desktop wallpaper.

PICT

PICT is the native graphics format for the Macintosh platform. It is the format used by system resources such as the Clipboard. PICT images can be opened by most Mac applications, including SimpleText.

Native Image-Editing Program Formats

Many image-editing programs use a proprietary file format that supports an editing feature called *layers*. The layers feature enables precise editing of various elements in a photograph, independent of other elements within the same image file. File formats that support this feature save the layers separately to allow further editing. These formats are lossless and can be quite large. Popular image-editing programs that support layers include Adobe Photoshop (*.psd), Adobe PhotoDeluxe (*.pdd), JASC Paint Shop Pro (*.psp), ArcSoft PhotoStudio (*.psf), and Ulead PhotoImpact (*.ufo).

Universal photo formats (such as TIFF and JPEG) do not support multiple layers. If you want to keep a copy of your image with the layers separate (that is, still available for independent editing), then you must save it in the photo editor's native format. If you decide to save the picture in another format such as TIFF or JPEG, the layers will automatically be merged into a single background layer during the save process.

Color Management

Ideally, the color you see reflected from a subject matches the color on the screen and in the final print. Maintaining color accuracy throughout the digital imaging process can be difficult and frustrating. Colors do not always reproduce as expected because of the different way in which input and output devices produce color (Fig. 8–9). Digital cameras, scanners, color monitors, televisions, and video projectors all create color through the additive color process by combining red, green, and blue light (RGB). Printers create color through the subtractive color process by combining cyan, magenta, yellow, and black (CMYK) inks or pigments on paper. The difference between these fundamental color reproduction methods accounts for much of the difficulty in maintaining color accuracy.

Compounding this issue are variations in how different input and output devices handle color. Different devices use different mixes of primary colors in an attempt to produce accurate color output. The specific range of color that a device can record, produce, or display is known as its *color gamut*. Generally speaking, RGB devices are capable of a wider color gamut than CMYK devices, and the color gamut of all printing and display systems is smaller than what the eye can perceive. Colors that fall outside the gamut of one of the devices in an imaging system will reproduce differently than expected.

Color management is the attempt to maintain color accuracy throughout the digital imaging chain by providing a communication framework between devices with differences in color gamut. Today's color management systems are

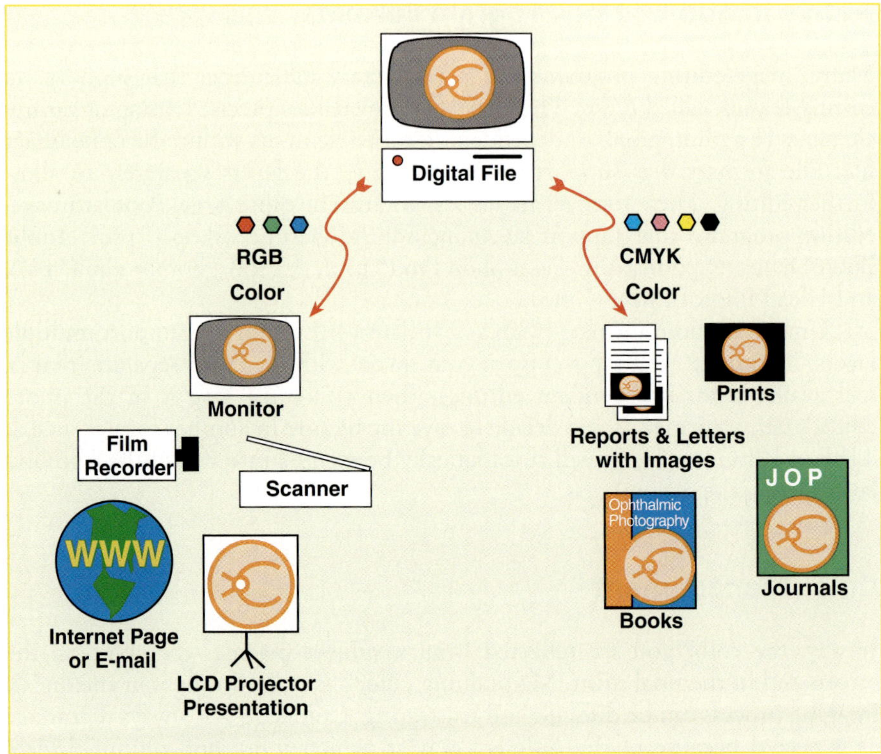

Figure 8–9 ○ Many color management issues are related to the fundamental differences between the additive (RGB) color system and the subtractive (CMYK) system. The additive system uses combinations of red, green, and blue light to create a full spectrum of colors. Monitors, projectors, cameras, and scanners use the additive system to create color with "light." The subtractive system is used for printed color output. Cyan, magenta, and yellow pigments are combined to absorb or "subtract" certain colors from white light illuminating the printed page. Black (K) is often added to the CMY mix to improve deep tone densities. Simply put, RGB devices start out with black and create color with light, while the CMYK process begins with a white surface and creates color by adding pigments.

based on the use of device color (ICC) profiles. These profiles describe how a device maps color to a universal color space that can be used by all devices and software programs in the imaging chain. The standard color space employed by most desktop imaging systems and peripheral devices is known as *sRGB*. For color management to work, a profile must be installed for each device in the system. Profiles for inkjet printers assume that a specific type of ink and a specific paper are being used. So make sure to use the correct paper settings when color reproduction is important. Using a calibrated monitor is also essential for predictable color output.

Recent versions of both Macintosh and Windows operating systems provide a basic, system-level color management system (ColorSync for Macintosh and Image Color Management for Windows 98, ME, 2000, and XP). System-level color management allows various programs to use the color management features of the operating system. An ICC profile, supplied by the hardware manufacturer, is loaded on installation of most new peripheral devices. This profile is typically used whenever colors are scanned, displayed, or printed.

Different programs and devices offer varying degrees of adjustment to color management preferences and monitor calibration. Many basic programs implement color management automatically and offer limited user adjustments. Some programs and scanner drivers will simply permit you to select the color management feature and specify a particular printer (and ICC profile). In Adobe Photo-Deluxe, for example, the command *Adjust Color Printing* can be found in the File menu. *Color Matching* can be selected under Preferences in VistaScan, the software driver for Umax scanners (Fig. 8–10). Other programs provide similar settings to enable basic color management.

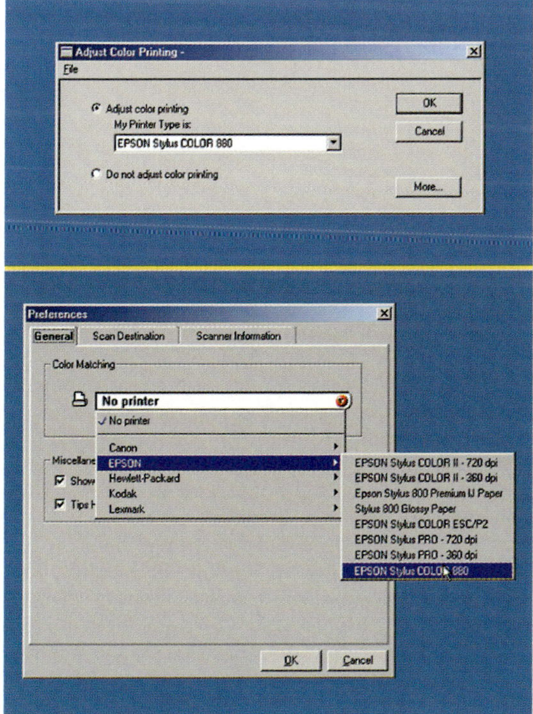

Figure 8–10 ○ Examples of basic color management controls provided with many entry-level graphics programs and imaging peripherals: *Top*, The "Adjust Color Printing" box used by Adobe PhotoDeluxe to select the color profile for a specific printer. *Bottom*, Use the "Preferences" dialog box to select your printer before scanning with Umax Vista-Scan software.

More advanced programs allow you to select a variety of color management settings, which may be helpful when printed images appear much different than expected. A common Windows interface, usually found under Preferences in the File menu, provides a check box to turn color management on or off (Fig. 8–11). When color management is selected, you can choose between *Basic*, an automatic setting, or *Proofing*. Proofing supplies a "soft-proof," in which the monitor emulates the color gamut of the output device (usually a printer). If you select the proofing option, you then need to select a rendering intent from the drop-down menu. Depending on the operating system, there may be different choices, but typically, they are *Perceptual, Relative Colorimetric, Saturation*, and *Absolute Colorimetric*. The rendering intents specify how color gamut differences are resolved between devices. Different intents work better than others depending on the type of image being printed. Perceptual is usually best for photographs. Experiment to find what works best for your system. High-end imaging and desktop publishing programs may offer more sophisticated color management controls (Fig. 8–12).

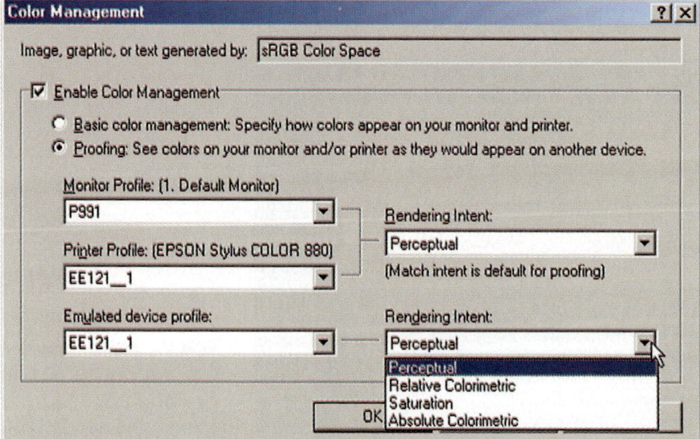

Figure 8–11 ○ If your graphics program supports Windows ICM color management, you can enable this feature and select preferences for device profiles and rendering intents. Device profiles communicate specific color characteristics to the color management system. Select the Enable Color Management check box, and try the Basic setting first. For more advanced control use the proofing option and select the *Perceptual* rendering intent for fundus photographs (and most other photographic images). This will allow you to preview (within the limitations of your monitor) how an image will look when printed on the specified printer. Other rendering intents include *Saturation, Relative Colorimetric*, and *Absolute Colorimetric. Saturation* is best for graphics in which color intensity is more important than accuracy. *Relative Colorimetric* is better for logos or other graphics with few colors that must be matched exactly. *Absolute Colorimetric* is used to map colors to a device-independent color space. In Windows 2000 and XP the same rendering intents are renamed *Pictures, Graphics, Proof,* and *Match.*

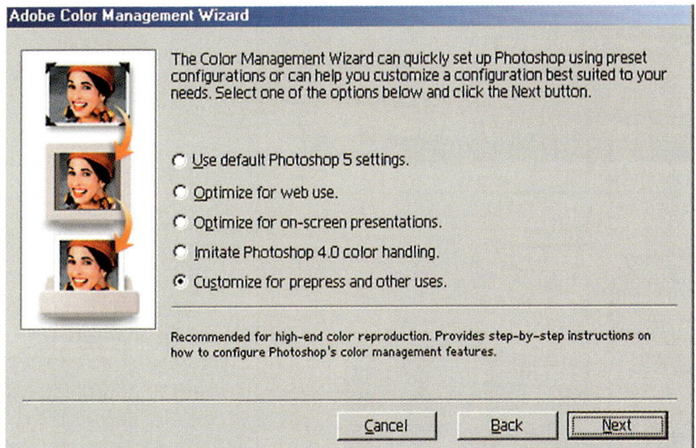

Figure 8–12 ◌ The Adobe Color Management Wizard will guide you through the process of configuring PhotoShop for accurate and reliable color reproduction. For this color management feature to be effective, calibrate your monitor first.

Monitor calibration is an important component of color management. Monitor settings for contrast, brightness, and color temperature will affect how an image appears on your screen. Using the ICC profile supplied with the monitor will not account for adjustments made to these settings. Calibration is necessary for critical color reproduction. Certain high-level imaging applications such as Adobe Photoshop and Corel PHOTO-PAINT supply a monitor calibration utility that helps you to balance your monitor's contrast, brightness, gamma, and white point to create a custom profile (Fig. 8–13).

If you find that colors are not printing as expected, there are a few things that you can check. First, if the printer supports ColorSync or ICM color management, you can enable this feature in your graphics program. Next, select similar color management settings in the printer driver. When you print on an inkjet printer, using good paper with the correct paper settings will go a long way toward ensuring reasonable color reproduction. If the printer does not support color management, make sure this feature is turned off in the imaging application.

When consistent, accurate color reproduction is essential, more sophisticated color management solutions might be necessary. The best color management systems require calibration of every device in the imaging chain. Calibration can be difficult and expensive. Results from custom device profiles are more accurate and reliable than the factory-installed profiles. This sophisticated level of color management is typically used in professional graphics, prepress, and publishing settings.

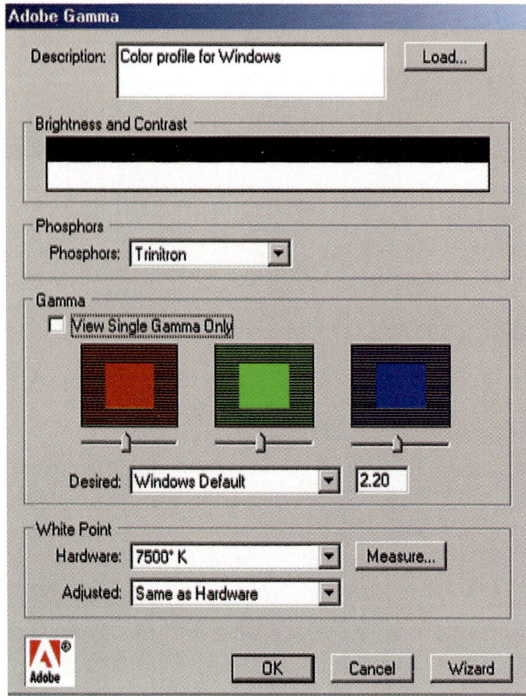

Figure 8–13 ◯ The Adobe Gamma dialog box allows you to adjust your monitor and create a personalized ICC profile. You can use the control panel shown here to adjust settings or use the step-by-step wizard to calibrate your monitor and define its color profile.

Resources

Books and Articles

Davies A: Digital Imaging A to Z. Boston: Butterworth-Heinemann, 2001.

Davies A, Fennessy P: Digital Imaging for Photographers, 4th Edition. Boston: Butterworth-Heinemann, 2001.

Fraser B: Color management explained. Photo Electronic Imaging 1998;41(5):30–35.

King JA: Digital Photography for Dummies, 3rd Edition. New York: Hungry Minds, 2000.

Rodney A: Resolution: An in-the-trenches guide to resolution basics. Photo Electronic Imaging 1998;4(2):38–44.

Rodney A: A gamut of solutions. Photo Electronic Imaging 1999;42(10):28–34.

Rodney A: Examining the new image file formats. Photo Electronic Imaging 2000;43(8):38.

Romano FJ: Delmar's Dictionary of Digital Printing and Publishing. Albany, NY: Delmar Publishers, 1997.

Web Sites

www.color.org
www.displaymate.com
www.dpcorner.com
www.extremetech.com
www.pantone.com
www.pcguide.com
www.pctechguide.com

Web Sites

www.color.org
www.displaymate.com
www.dpcorner.com
www.extremetech.com
www.pantone.com
www.pcguide.com
www.pctechguide.com

Chapter 9

Digital Image Capture

The first (and most obvious) step in the digital imaging chain is to get retinal images into a computer. This chapter describes the various ways in which fundus photographs can be digitized, including direct image capture and scanning.

Direct Capture

The easiest way to acquire digital fundus images is through direct capture using a fundus camera that is equipped for high-resolution digital imaging. Early digital systems consisted of a CCD video camera coupled to a digitizing board in the computer to convert the analog video signal to digital. The latest generation of digital cameras perform the analog-to-digital conversion in the camera itself, eliminating the need for an external digitizing board or frame grabber. Digital capture devices have been adapted to many traditional mydriatic fundus camera models for color fundus photography as well as fluorescein and indocyanine green (ICG) angiography.

A number of ophthalmic camera manufacturers and third-party vendors offer digital solutions for ophthalmic imaging. Canon, Kowa, Topcon/Imagenet, and Zeiss are major ophthalmic instrument manufacturers that provide complete digital imaging systems adapted to their traditional, film-capable fundus cameras. Third-party vendors such as Ophthalmic Imaging Systems (OIS), MRP Group, Escalon Medical Imaging (EMI), and Eye Expert offer custom-imaging solutions that are retrofitted to new or existing fundus camera models. Commercially produced digital fundus imaging systems are complete solutions. They supply tools for all steps of the digital imaging process: capture, processing, storage, retrieval, and display.

Depending on the CCD camera configuration, image resolution in current retinal imaging systems varies from 800 × 600 up to 3000 × 2000 pixels. As manufacturers have moved from video-based electronic cameras to true digital sensors, image quality has improved. When matched with fundus cameras that exhibit high optical resolution, current 3k × 2k capture devices produce images that rival the quality of 35-mm film. Increased bit depth (10 or 12 bits per color) also improves image quality by increasing exposure latitude and highlight detail, especially in the optic nerve.

Nonmydriatic fundus cameras with digital capture capabilities are often used as screening devices for diabetic retinopathy and glaucoma (some units still use video cameras). These cameras utilize a video-based viewing/illumination system that adapts well to digital capture. Current models from Topcon, Nidek, and Canon feature USB output or removable storage devices like Compact Flash cards to aid in transferring images from the capture device to a computer. Topcon's TRC-NW6S nonmydriatic camera is compatible with IMAGEnet MOSAIC software, which allows the stitching together of multiple images to create a retinal montage from up to nine fields of view.

For many years, the trend has been to adapt digital technology to fundus cameras originally designed and equipped with 35-mm or Polaroid film backs. More recently, new instruments have been developed which rely entirely on digital capture technology. These new digital-only cameras include the RetCam 120 from Massie Research Laboratories, the NM-100D from Nidek, and the Digital Fundus Imager from OIS. The RetCam 120 is a digital-only fundus camera designed for wide-field imaging of pediatric eyes (Fig. 9–1). It utilizes a portable hand-held capture unit that is tethered to a computer console. Interchangeable diagnostic contact lenses are available in 120-degree, 130-degree, and 30-degree fields of view. The optics and light delivery system of this specialized instrument are optimized for the pediatric eye, which limits the camera use to children and young adults. The NM-100D (see Fig. 1–15 on page 14) from Nidek is a portable, noncontact, handheld nonmydriatic digital camera with standard video-out for connection to a video printer. The OIS Digital Fundus Imager (Fig. 9–2) utilizes live-motion digital video technology for fundus imaging without the need for flash illumination. Images are saved in the motion JPEG format. The next generation of fundus cameras will likely include more digital-only models.

Images acquired by direct capture can be enhanced, printed, archived, retrieved, and exported by using the proprietary imaging application that is supplied with the digital system. Images from a photographic session are available instantly and are typically displayed in a proof sheet or thumbnail image format. Images can then be viewed or printed individually or in groups (including a "4-up" or "9-up"). Commercially produced fundus imaging systems may include measurement tools calibrated to the magnification of the fundus camera to provide accurate tracking of lesion size (Fig. 9–3).

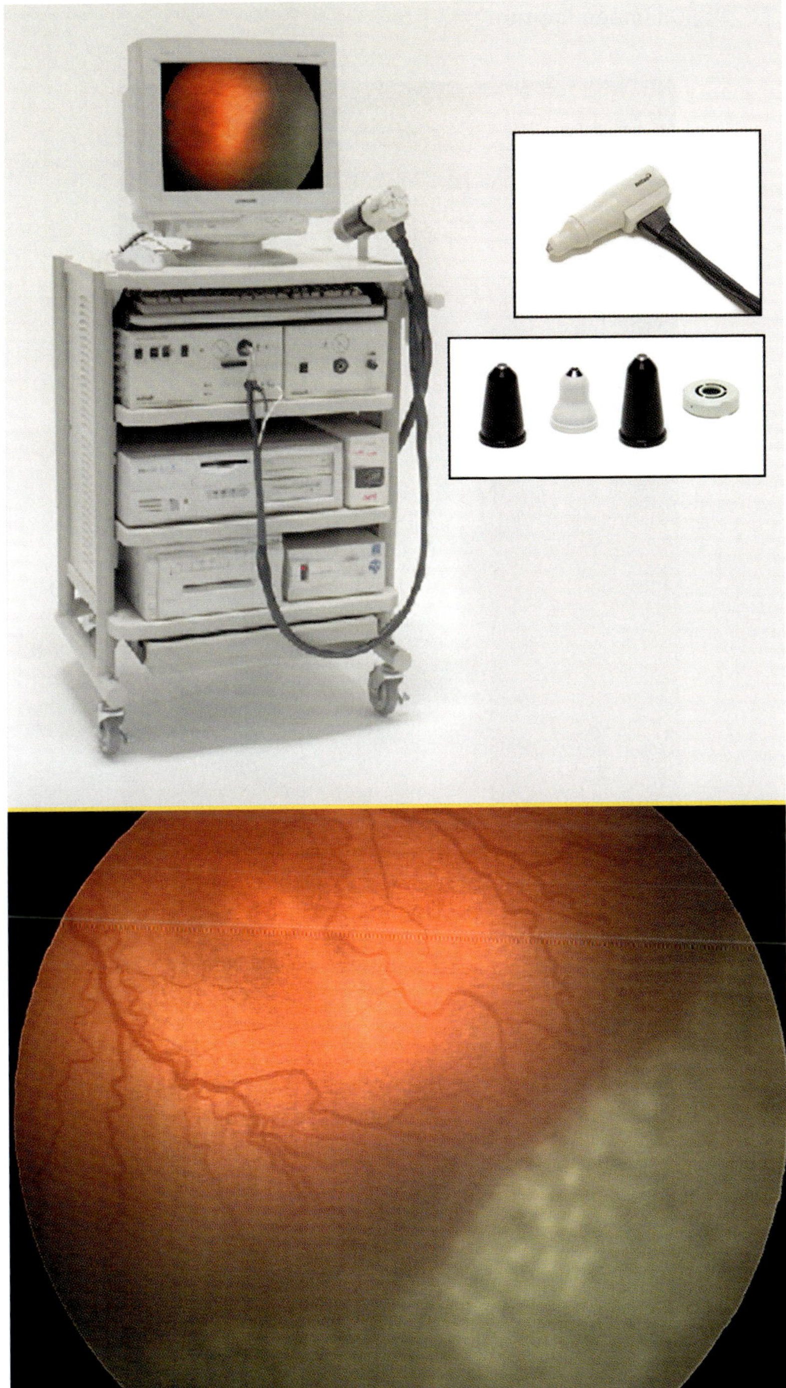

Figure 9–1 ○ *Top*, The RetCam 120 system is composed of multiple components on a mobile cart, including a monitor, keyboard, and mouse; a hand-held image capture unit with a 3CCD video camera; and interchangeable lenses or "nosepieces." (Courtesy Massie Research, Dublin, California.) *Bottom*, RetCam image of peripheral laser treatment for retinopathy of prematurity (ROP).

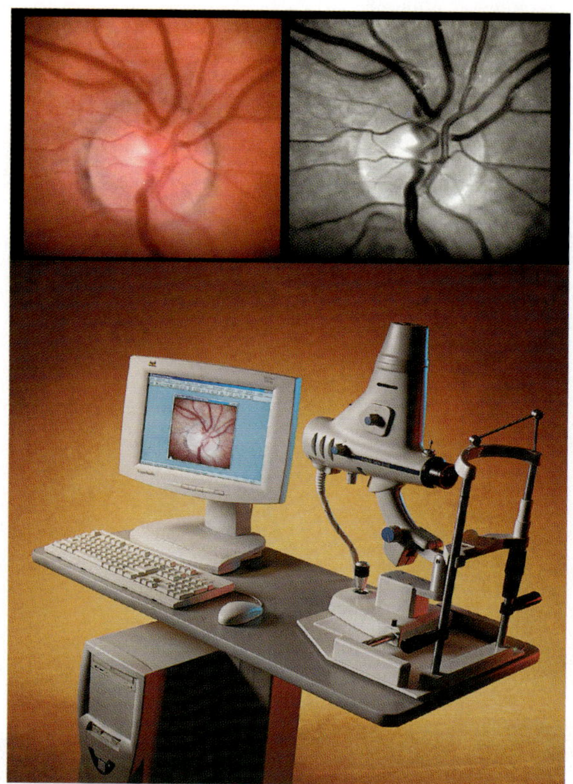

Figure 9–2 ○ The OIS Digital Fundus Imager II is an all-digital retinal camera that captures live-motion fundus images in color or black and white. This system can also be used to capture real-time fluorescein angiography and can be equipped with an option to perform ICG feeder-vessel angiography. (Image courtesy of Ophthalmic Imaging Systems, Sacramento, CA.)

The enhancement tools that are supplied with these systems will allow changes to the brightness, contrast, sharpness, and color balance of images being displayed or printed. For medical record purposes, it is vital that we retain the integrity of the original image. This is an important issue in using digital imaging because an original digital image, unlike the traditional film image, can be easily modified. Enhanced images can be added to the patient's record, but the original image files should be stored without modification. Whether you are using a digital image system or keeping your own set of electronic patient files, make sure that the original file is not overwritten when enhancements are made.

The owner's manual for each digital system will have specific instructions describing how to export images from the imaging software to an imaging file

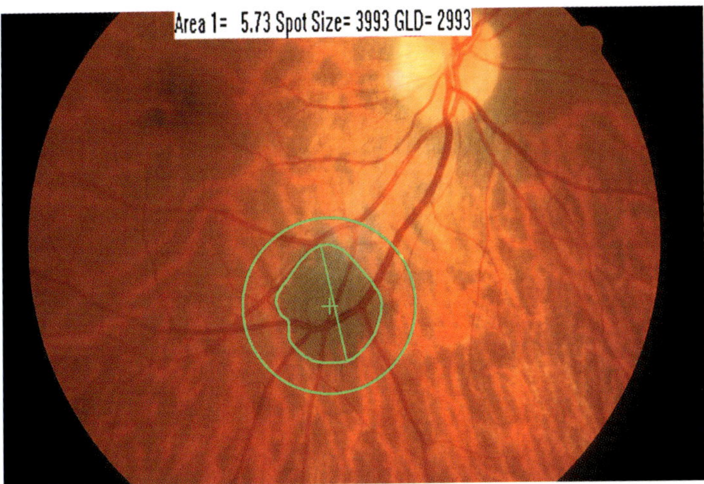

Figure 9–3 ○ OIS WinStation Area Measure tool used to outline and measure a choroidal nevus. Before using this tool for the first time, follow the manufacturer's instructions on calibration for your specific fundus camera at each angle of view. Use the mouse to place points on the lesion margins. Once the outline is complete, the computer calculates the total area and greatest linear dimension. Although this tool was designed to facilitate measurement of choroidal neovascular membranes for photodynamic therapy (PDT), it can be used to measure other lesion types. The outer ring represents the recommended treatment area for PDT.

folder or a separate disk. Generally, you will use the Download, Export, or Save As command. You may be able to choose a specific file type (for example, .tif or .jpg), and you will be asked to navigate to the folder or disk in which you would like to place the copy of the image.

Off-the-shelf digital hardware and software are constantly improving in quality and ease of use. It can be tempting to adapt these products to a traditional fundus camera to create a do-it-yourself digital system.[1] Professional-grade single-lens reflex (SLR) digital camera backs with large-capacity storage cards will fit the camera mounts on certain fundus camera models. Before attempting to attach a digital camera back to a fundus camera, there are a number of technical issues that you should consider. The physical size of the imaging chip in many digital camera backs is usually smaller than the size of 35-mm film and results in cropping of the fundus image. When full-size chips become more common, this cropping effect will be eliminated. Digital camera backs can be sensitive to flash voltage discrepancies when connected to an external flash source like a fundus camera. It is important to follow the manufacturer's recommendations on flash trigger circuit voltages to avoid potential damage to the camera back. You will also need to consider how you will view images during capture and review. If your camera has a video-out connection, you can view images on a video monitor. If not, you may be limited to the small LCD screen on the camera back, making it difficult to judge focus and illumination until you transfer images to a computer.

The method of file handling and retrieval is another important consideration in developing your own system. There are a number of programs that will enable to you to track and retrieve image files. (See the section on image file management later in this chapter.) For high-volume clinical use, the image-capture software and robust database supplied with a vendor-produced system are often the best software solution. Technical support is another advantage of the vendor-produced solution, and many users opt for the security and reliability of these systems. We may soon see the emergence of software solutions that will facilitate the integration of these camera backs. Until that time, we do not recommend the build-your-own solution for routine clinical use unless you are comfortable troubleshooting technical issues on your own.

Scanning

Next to direct digital capture, scanners are probably the easiest way to acquire digital fundus photographs. Scanners can be used for both reflective and transparent image media (including prints, slides, and X-rays). There are three main types of scanners:

- Professional drum scanners, which are capable of scanning both reflective art and transparencies at very high resolutions. They are typically used for prepress preparation of images by publishing houses. They cost tens of thousands of dollars.
- Home/office desktop flatbed scanners designed to scan documents, photos, or flat objects. Some flatbed scanners have document feed mechanisms that allow unattended scanning of multiple sheets or transparent material adapters that allow scanning of slides and negatives (Fig. 9–4).
- Dedicated film scanners, which pass light through an image. The optics and scan head are maximized for the small size associated with different film formats.

Scanners typically utilize charge-coupled devices (CCD) similar to those used in video and digital still cameras. The CCD sensors are arranged in a long, thin row and record light that is reflected from (or transmitted through) the original photograph. The number of CCD elements in this row will determine the optical resolution of the x-direction. The scanner's light source moves across the scanning bed in synchronization with the scanning head. A stepping motor moves the CCD array across the scanning bed in very small, precise increments to achieve the y-direction scanning rate.

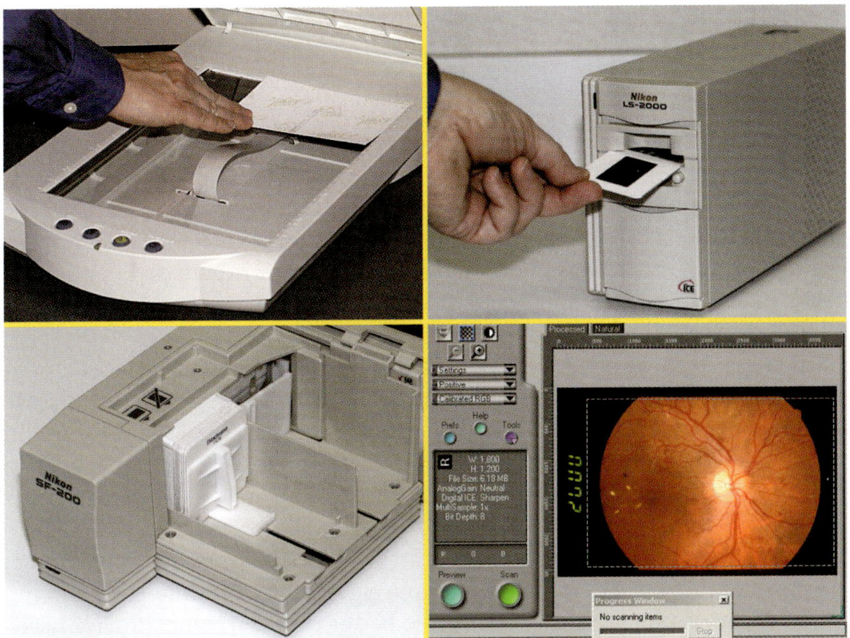

Figure 9–4 ○ *Upper left,* Desktop flatbed scanner in use. *Upper right,* Film scanners can be used to scan slides or negatives at resolutions up to 4000 ppi. *Lower left,* Optional automatic slide feed mechanism for unattended batch scanning of up to 50 slides. *Lower right,* The image preview window shows crop selection and scanner settings.

Scanners connect to a computer in a variety of ways to transfer data: SCSI, parallel port, USB, and FireWire/IEEE 1394. For a number of years, SCSI (Small Computer System Interface) was the standard. SCSI is built into most Macintosh computers but requires the installation of a SCSI card in a PC, which sometimes can be complicated. More recently, USB has become the connection interface of choice. It features plug-and-play technology that is compatible with newer operating systems such as Windows 98, ME, 2000, and XP and MacOS 8.1 or greater. Most computers, scanners, and printers manufactured today have USB ports installed. This has made scanner installation and setup easier and provides a faster transfer rate than parallel port. FireWire/IEEE 1394 is a high-performance peripheral standard with a fast data-transfer rate that makes it ideal for transferring large files from high-end digital cameras, video cameras, and scanners. FireWire connections are standard on most Macs and some PCs. USB 2.0 is a new standard with transfer speeds that rival FireWire. Although the data-transfer rates are up to 40 times faster than USB, the memory buffer in most scanners may be too small to take full advantage of high-speed transfer.

The slight increase in scanning speed with FireWire and USB 2.0 scanners is an advantage in high-volume settings.

Scanner Selection

Since most film-based fundus photography is shot on 35-mm transparency film, scanning slides is a very common practice. Film scanners are an excellent way to digitize high-quality fundus photographs from slides or negatives. Film originals possess higher resolution and greater dynamic range than photographic prints, and film scanners are designed to record this extra detail.

If you need to scan Polaroid prints from a nonmydriatic camera, you might require a flatbed scanner. Some flatbed scanners are equipped with a transparent media adapter or filmstrip adapter that will allow the scanning of 35-mm film. Today's flatbed scanners, with optical resolutions of 1200 ppi and higher, are adequate for occasional low- or medium-quality scans from film. The filmstrip adapters will eliminate the Newton rings that are often associated with imaging film pressed against a glass surface. Scanners with an optical resolution of 600 ppi (the standard just a few years ago) do not do a good job of scanning 35-mm film.

A dedicated film scanner remains the better choice if your primary need is scanning slides. This is especially true in a high-volume setting, in which many images may need to be digitized at medium or high resolution. Film scanners typically boast a maximum optical scanning resolution of 2000–4000 ppi. High-resolution capability is important in scanning film because of the amount of scaling needed to enlarge the film original. The software interface and controls work very much as they do on a flatbed scanner, but scaling becomes more important since the 35-mm film has an image area of 1.5×1 inches or less. For example, scanning a 35-mm slide or negative for printing at 6×9 inches would require linear scaling by 600%. Film scanner software typically provides a scaling calculator, which allows you to easily size the image for printing while scanning. Nikon, Minolta, Polaroid, Canon, and Microtek all make high-quality film scanners.

There is a wide range of models to choose from, in both cost and quality. Scanners use prisms, lenses, and mirrors to direct light to the CCD array. A high-quality scanner will use high-quality, color-corrected glass optics, while inexpensive models may use plastic components to reduce costs. Better scanners also use high-grade, low-noise electronics to improve image quality. Be sure to compare the optical (rather than interpolated) resolution specifications. Software drivers and scanning interfaces vary widely as well, so choose carefully on the basis of the software tools that are best for your situation. Low-end scanner software will emphasize automatic image adjustment, while better-quality programs will offer powerful, more adjustable tools. Connectivity is another important consideration. Make sure that your computer will support the data transfer method used by the scanner you are considering. Some film scanners accept accessory batch feeders that will scan up to 50 slides in a session as long as the slide mounts are not warped or dog-eared from handling.

A number of manufacturers offer 36-, 42-, or 48-bit models that can scan images at higher bit depth. High-bit-depth scanning results in increased dynamic range, which can reduce noise and improve detail in shadows and/or highlights. This capability is more important in film scanners, since film originals possess greater dynamic range than reflective originals. Very few software programs can handle expanded-bit-depth image files, and most monitors and digital output devices are limited to 24-bit output, so high-bit-depth capture might not always be as useful as it sounds. These scanners will usually compress high-bit-depth scans and save the image file in 24-bit color. If you use an imaging program that accepts high bit-depth image files, you will notice a significant increase in file size and memory required.

Certain models supply a digital dust-removal feature that can reduce dust spots, scratches, and fingerprints on the original image. This is especially helpful in scanning slides or negatives (Fig. 9–5). Digital dust removal utilizes an infrared scanning channel to identify dust and scratches. The infrared scan is compared with the visible light data, and the artifacts are overwritten with interpolated pixels. This feature works quite well but slows the scanning process and results in a reduction of image sharpness. Unfortunately, the dust-removal feature will not work with black-and-white or Kodachrome films because these emulsions block infrared transmission. You can still scan these film types; just make sure to turn the dust-removal feature off.

Scanning Techniques

Use the following step-by-step approach to scanning for repeatable results (Table 9–1).

1. **Start the scanner software.** Start the scanner software program or a TWAIN-compliant application such as Photoshop, and activate the scanner driver by selecting it as the active TWAIN source in the File menu (see the accompanying box, "Twain Standards.") Reset the scanner to the default settings. Some scanning drivers will allow you to save user-defined settings that are useful for frequently performed scanning tasks.
2. **Set the scan mode.** Set the scan mode to match the image type. For most color fundus photographs, this mode would be 24-bit color. If the original image is a black-and-white photograph, then gray-scale mode is appropriate. *Line art* setting would be used for high-contrast black-and-white scans, and *text* setting for optical character recognition.

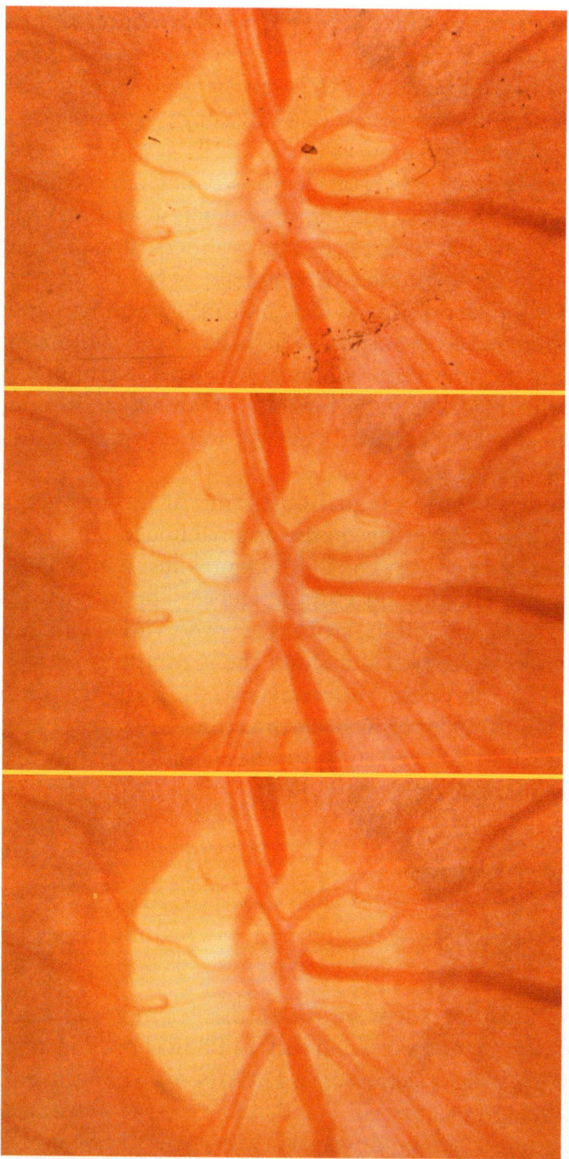

Figure 9–5 ○ *Top*, High-magnification view of a dusty slide. *Center*, Digital dust removal utilizes an extra scanning pass with an infrared light source to create a defect channel that identifies artifacts such as dust and scratches. Any pixels that are identified by the scanning software as dust artifacts are removed and replaced with interpolated pixels. *Bottom*, Final "clean" image after sharpening.

Table 9–1 **Scanning, Step by Step**
1. Start the software driver, and reset to default settings. 2. Set the scan mode. 3. Set the film type to positive or negative. 4. Perform a preview scan. 5. Select or crop to the desired area. 6. Set the resolution and scaling. 7. Adjust the black and white points. 8. Set the midtones to the desired brightness. 9. Select the Descreen filter if necessary. 10. Select the desired sharpen filter. 11. Perform the scan. 12. Save the image in the appropriate file format.

3. **Set the film type.** When scanning film originals, set the film type selector to positive or negative to match the original. The color negative mode will compensate for the orange mask that is used in common color negative films.

4. **Preview the scan.** Place the photo on the scanning bed, and perform a preview scan. A low-resolution image will appear in the preview area.

5. **Crop.** Use the selection tool to size the scan area to fit the image being scanned. Cropping before the scan eliminates unwanted areas and maintains a practical file size. You can also crop afterward, in an image-editing program, but capturing a larger area than needed will cause you and the computer to work harder than necessary.

TWAIN Standards

The TWAIN standard is an image data transfer protocol that allows one software package to recognize input from multiple devices such as scanners and digital cameras. Scanning through a TWAIN-compliant application is usually preferable to using the scanner driver as a stand-alone application. Once scanning is complete, the scanner driver hands the image off to an active window in the TWAIN-compliant application. Many common word-processing, desktop publishing, and graphics applications support the TWAIN standard, so you can scan directly into the application you are using.

Unlike most other computer terms, TWAIN is not an acronym. The name that was originally chosen was already trademarked, so the programmers found last-minute inspiration in the saying "Never the twain shall meet." Contrary to popular folklore, TWAIN does not stand for "Technology Without An Interesting Name."

6. **Set the resolution.** One of the most important rules of scanning is to match the scanning resolution to the resolution of the intended output device. While you might be tempted to scan at the highest resolution, it is far more practical to match the scanning resolution with output resolution (Table 9–2). Today's scanners have optical resolution that may be more than necessary for many common image uses. When full optical resolution is unnecessary, we suggest scanning at a resolution that is an even divisor of the true optical resolution of the scanner. For example, if the scanner's optical resolution is 1200 ppi, then scanning at settings such as 600 ppi, 300 ppi, and 150 ppi is preferable to scanning at 720 ppi, 360 ppi, and so on. The idea is that the scanner software has an easier time resampling these evenly divisible numbers of pixels to achieve the desired resolution. You can also resample later, in an image-editing program with the help of the computer, which has more robust processing capabilities than the scanner firmware. For this reason, some professionals prefer to do any resampling in a high-quality image editor such as Adobe Photoshop.

Table 9–2
Scan for Intended Use

Output Resolution Intended use	Suggested resolution starting points in pixels per inch (ppi) or pixel dimensions	Approximate size of uncompressed .tif (final .jpg will be smaller)
Web display	72–150 ppi at screen size	0.5–2.25 MB
E-mail (screen display)	72–150 ppi at screen size	0.5–2.25 MB
PowerPoint (screen display)	72–150 ppi scaled to maximum frame size 7.5 × 10 inches	1.1–4.75 MB
Dye-sublimation printer (true 300 dpi)	300 ppi	9 MB
Inkjet printer (photo-quality output on photo paper)	150–300 ppi or printer dpi setting divided by 3.	4-9 MB
Referral letter (plain paper)	150 ppi	2 MB
Film recorder (set at 4k output resolution)	Pixel dimensions: 4096 × 2731 or 2048 × 1366	15 MB or 8 MB
Publication in journal or text	Twice the lines per inch of publication. Usually 150 lpi × 2 = 300 ppi.	9 MB

Screen resolution varies by the type of monitor and settings being used. In scanning for screen display, it is useful to think in terms of pixel dimensions rather than pixels per inch because the number of pixels per inch is somewhat irrelevant. For example, a 4 × 6 photograph scanned at 100 ppi will result in an image with pixel dimensions of 600 × 400. This image will nearly fill the screen on a VGA monitor (640 × 480 display). The same image will fill less than half the screen area of an XGA monitor (1024 × 768 display). If the screen resolution of the intended monitor or video projector is known ahead of time, the scan resolution can be set to match. If the image will be distributed or displayed on multiple monitors of varying sizes and resolution standards, then using the lowest common denominator of VGA resolution makes sense. (See Table 8–1 for a list of monitor resolution standards.) Images that are intended for display on the World Wide Web are typically limited to 640 × 480 for this reason.

The most practical resolution for images you wish to e-mail will vary depending on the final use of the image. If the images are intended for screen viewing, keep the resolution low and the file size small. If the e-mail recipient will print or publish the image, then use a setting that matches

What Resolution to Use When You Do Not Know the Intended Output

It is always best to know what pixel dimensions or page size is needed for final output, but there may be times when you need to scan an image without knowing how it will eventually be used. We often get requests from colleagues to scan fundus images that will be used "later." This is a common scenario in using a batch scanner to scan multiple slides from a teaching collection for archiving or for future presentation or publication purposes. When faced with this situation, try to determine the maximum resolution you are likely to need.

Commercial printing generally requires high-resolution images, so if there is any chance the image will be published, scan with enough resolution to produce a good print: 300 ppi at the maximum print size. For an 8 × 10-inch print, this means an image of 2400 × 3000 pixels for an uncompressed file size of 20 MB. Scanning images at this size may be impractical (especially if you are scanning numerous images) and will result in far more resolution than you will need for most purposes.

A good compromise is to scan at pixel dimensions of approximately 1200 × 1800. This results in an uncompressed file size of just over 6 MB. You can save the image in a lossless file format or compress it as a high-quality JPEG file (200–300KB final file size) after making any necessary corrections to brightness, contrast, and color balance. This results in a print size of 4 × 6 inches at 300 ppi and provides more than enough resolution for most publication or screen display purposes. If it is a particularly valuable photograph and you have only one opportunity to capture as much detail as you can, scan at 2000 × 3000. But for routine use, 1200 × 1800 is a practical guideline.

the resolution of the recipient's output device, and compress the file for transfer by using the JPEG format.

Choosing a scanning resolution for inkjet printing is based on the printer settings and paper type you will use. A general rule of thumb is to scan at 25–33% of the printer's dpi output. Scan a photo at approximately 120 ppi when adding the image to a referral letter being printed on plain paper at a printer setting of 360 dpi. For photo-quality output on good paper at 1200 to 1440 dpi settings, scan the original image at approximately 300–400 ppi.

Scan for publication at twice the lines per inch (lpi) of the imagesetter used by the publisher. Many professional journals use a line screen setting of 150 lpi, so good results can be obtained by scaling the image to actual publication size at a resolution setting of 300 ppi.

If you are scanning photographic prints, you can scan at actual size using an appropriate resolution (in ppi) for the intended output device. Film originals are typically enlarged for output, so it may be more practical to use pixel dimensions to determine resolution in scanning slides or negatives. Otherwise, scaling will set the intended output size at an appropriate resolution in pixels per inch. Keep in mind that the quality of the original photograph will also have an effect on resolution. Color photographic prints might not be capable of showing a noticeable quality difference at any setting over 200 ppi. The practical limit may be 150 ppi for scans from texts or journals.

7. **Adjust the black point and white point.** Prescan tonal corrections maximize image quality by adjusting brightness and contrast. Postscanning tonal adjustments can also be made in an image-editing program, but good-quality scans are easier to work with, so it pays to get as much tonal quality as possible when scanning. Low-end scanners often have limited tools for adjusting tonal quality, usually emphasizing automatic adjustment. Automatic adjustments may work well with average pictures that contain multiple colors and equal amounts of light and dark tones. Applying this type of correction to a typical fundus photograph, however, may have an unintended detrimental effect on quality. The autocorrection is likely to adjust the color balance to "correct" the orange bias from fundus pigmentation and increase overall exposure to compensate for the black mask surrounding the image. The resulting overcorrected scan will likely be too light, with poor saturation and incorrect (greenish-blue) color balance (Fig. 9–6).

Better scanning programs supply various tools for setting the black, white, and midtone levels that offer greater flexibility than autoadjustments. Depending on the specific scanning program, these adjustment tools may be called Histogram, Levels, or Curves. Using one of these features is preferable

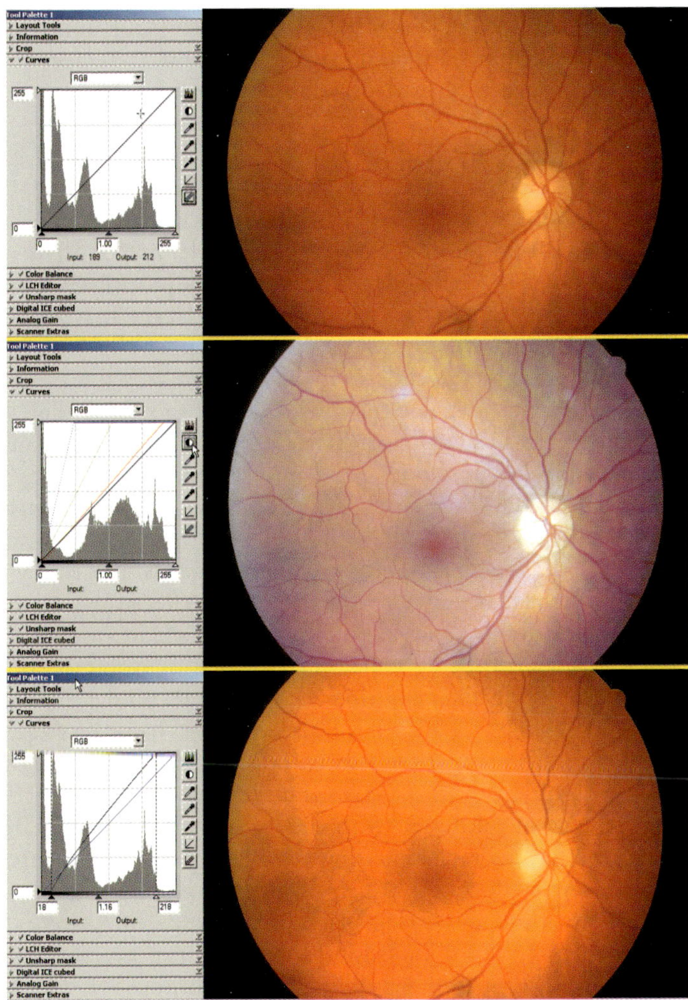

Figure 9–6 ○ The automatic image-adjustment controls that are provided with many scanners usually do not work well on fundus photographs owing to the high concentration of red/yellow colors and the lack of true highlights. *Top,* Uncorrected scan of fundus image with accompanying histogram. *Center,* Scanned image with autocorrection applied. Note the overexposure and color shift. *Bottom,* The same image adjusted visually with the aid of the histogram.

to using simple contrast and brightness tools. The contrast and brightness tools may discard data indiscriminately by applying global changes to the entire image. Using a histogram or curves tool allows you to decide which image data is changed or discarded. A histogram is a graph that displays the distribution of pixels for each brightness level in an image. You can use this graph to make informed decisions on how to maximize the tonal quality of an image.

The first step is to adjust shadow and highlight values by setting the black point and white point. Setting the black point determines level 0, or the darkest point on the brightness scale. The white point determines the pixels that will be set at the brightest white, or level 255. To set the black point, move the left-hand slider to the first group of pixels where values begin to rise. Then move the right-hand slider to the first group of pixel values on the right to set the white point or upper clip limit. Any pixel values to the right of the slider will be changed to white. Setting these points will effectively increase the tonal range of the image (Fig. 9–7).

Some programs use an Eyedropper tool to sample a group of pixels to set the black point, white point, and midtone values. A Curves tool may also be available. Unlike the Levels tool, Curves is not limited to just shadow, midtone, and highlight values; it will allow precise tonal correction by enabling the adjustment of multiple groups of pixels. It is a very powerful image adjustment tool that takes practice to use effectively.

8. **Adjust the midtones.** Once the highlight and shadow values have been set, the midtones can be lightened or darkened by using the midtone or gamma slider. Using this tool does not affect all pixel values, since the shadow and highlight values have already been defined. Adjusting the tonal values in this manner is a standard procedure in scanning that works well in a wide variety of image types. Fundus photos generally consist of a high percentage of midtones, with the exception of the black mask surrounding the fundus image. Setting the black point will ensure that the mask is a deep black. (This is helpful in later editing steps if you want to remove the mask by setting black as a transparent color.) Using the histogram may not always be helpful for setting the "correct" white point because of the lack of true highlights in many fundus images. When this happens, set the white point visually, or use the contrast and brightness tools to adjust the tonal range.

9. **Descreen.** Continuous-tone images scanned from publications often exhibit an unwanted effect called a moiré pattern (Fig. 9–8). The moiré pattern is caused by interference between the dot pattern of the scanner and the halftone dot pattern used for offset printing. The Descreen filter is used to minimize this pattern. A Descreen filter can usually be adjusted to match the print quality of the original image, expressed in lines per inch (lpi).

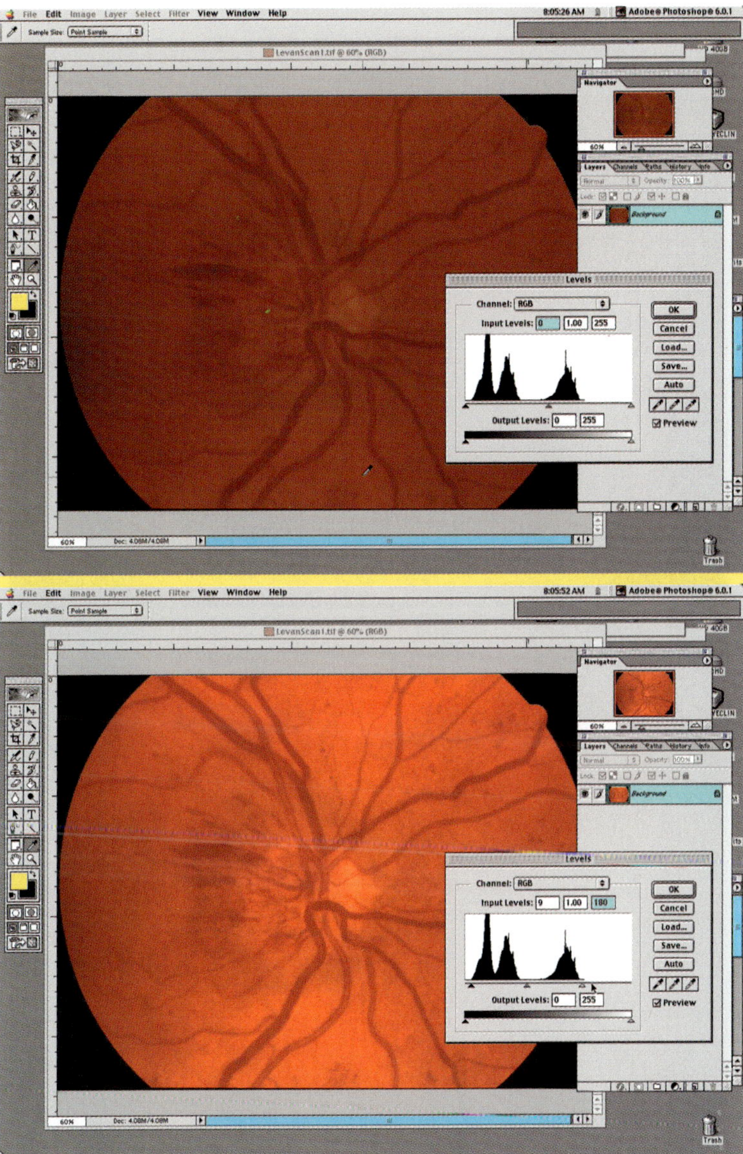

Figure 9–7 ○ Settings levels in most scanning programs is similar to using the Photoshop Levels tool shown here. *Top,* The original image is too dark and lacks contrast. The histogram shows a lack of pixel values on the right side of the scale. *Bottom,* The levels sliders have been adjusted to improve image brightness and contrast. First, the left-hand slider was moved to the right, to set the black level at the point where the pixel count begins to increase. Then the right-hand slider was shifted left, to set the highlight value at the point where pixel values begin to rise on the histogram. After the black and white points are set in this manner, the midtone slider can be used to adjust overall brightness.

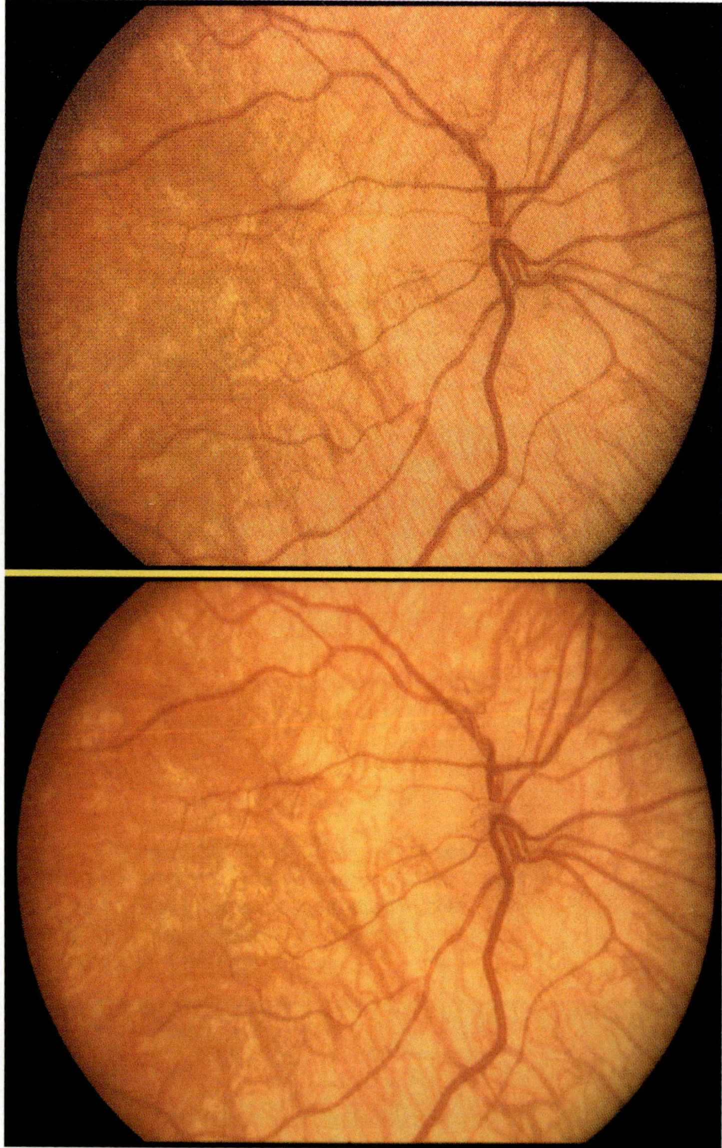

Figure 9–8 ○ *Top,* Image scanned from a printed publication demonstrating a moiré pattern caused by interference between the offset-printed halftone pattern and the pixel pattern of the scanner's CCD. *Bottom,* The same image scanned with a Descreen filter set at the appropriate line screen setting.

Newspapers typically print at 85 lpi, magazines at 133 lpi, journals and textbooks at 150 lpi, and high-quality art books at 175–200 lpi. Set the Descreen filter to match the type of original to smooth out the moiré pattern. This type of preprocessing will increase the scanning time considerably. Descreen tools are also available in most image-editing packages and can be applied after scanning has been completed. Make sure to leave this control off when it is not needed, as it reduces image sharpness.

10. **Sharpen.** Most scanned images appear a little soft and will benefit from the judicious use of a sharpening filter to increase apparent edge sharpness. This enhancement can be applied at capture or later, in an image-editing program. Most scanning applications provide only a very small preview window that makes it difficult to judge the degree of sharpening until the scan has been completed, and applying this filter will increase scanning time. If you are scanning at low resolution for e-mail, screen display, or direct importing into PowerPoint, then sharpen the image during the scan. Otherwise, save sharpening for later. Be careful not to oversharpen, as this can introduce undesirable noise in an image (Fig. 9–9).

11. **Scan.** Press the scan button on the screen. If you are scanning at a high resolution or are scanning multiple slides, go get a cup of coffee.

12. **Check the results.** Inspect the results after the scan is complete. If the image is acceptable, save the image to the desired location in an appropriate file format. (See Chapter 8 for a discussion of file formats.)

Other Image Acquisition Methods

When digital fundus cameras or scanners are unavailable, there are other ways to get fundus images into a computer. Many traditional photo-finishing labs offer scanning services as an option when color films are processed or printed. Kodak developed the Photo CD format for this purpose. A Photo CD features multiple versions of each image at various resolution settings and saved as an "Image Pac." When you access your images from a Photo CD, you can choose the image resolution that suits your output needs. Many imaging programs will open Kodak's proprietary file format (*.pcd), and the images can be edited and saved in different file formats such as JPEG or TIFF. If you do not have access to a high-quality scanner or need only occasional digital fundus images, this may be a good option to consider. It is important to note that some photo labs will apply automatic color and exposure correction to images while scanning. For consumer images, these corrections often improve the overall image quality, but fundus images will be overcorrected. If you are using a photo lab to scan fundus images to a Photo CD, you can ask them to scan without correction to prevent unwanted color shifts. Do not confuse the high-resolution scanning of the Photo

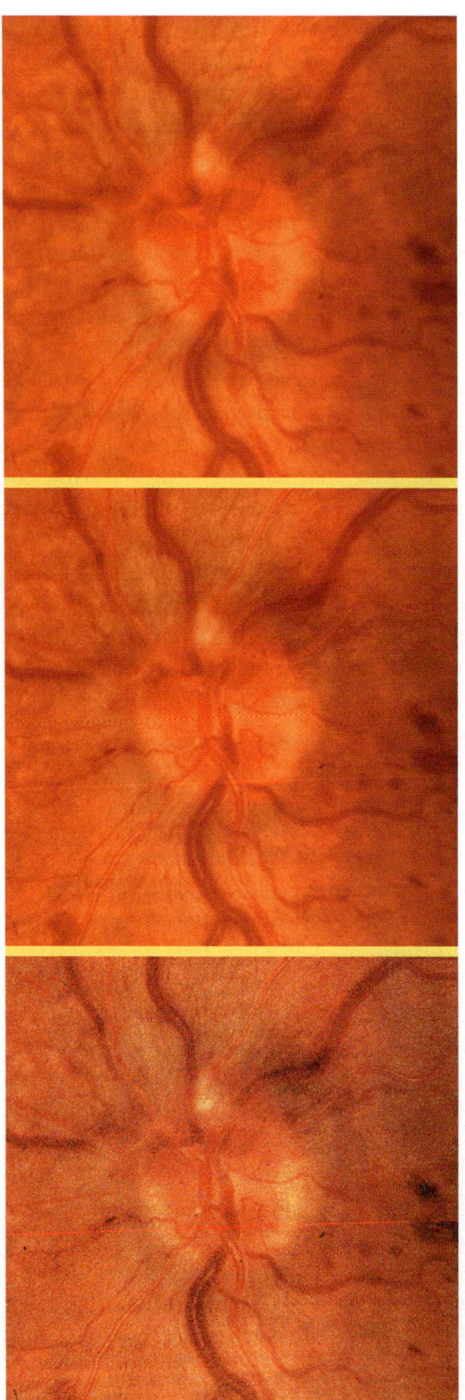

Figure 9–9 ○ *Top*, Scanned images often appear a little "soft" or out of focus. *Center*, Image scanned with a sharpening filter applied to improve apparent detail. *Bottom*, Oversharpening can result in excessive noise and degradation of the image. Sharpening is often applied after scanning, in an image-editing program with the Unsharp Mask filter, which offers greater control over this effect.

CD format with low-resolution scans offered by some processing labs. The Picture Disk format will fit up to 28 low-resolution compressed pictures on a 1.4 MB floppy disk. The image quality of these scans will be adequate for e-mail but not for medical purposes. Kodak also offers a Picture CD service, which includes scans at a single resolution (1024×1536) from color negative film (but not slides), at the time of processing only.

Telemedicine services offer another means of acquiring and sharing fundus photographs. The OcuNet Database is an example of a telemedicine service that utilizes standard web browsers to access ophthalmic images in a secure database (Fig. 9–10). With the correct password, users can access the image database from any location that has Internet access. Security is maintained through the use of Secure Socket Layers, the type of data encryption that is used to protect online banking transactions. OcuNet leases this database service to users with digital images, film originals, or a combination of both. You can upload images to the web server, or OcuNet (or other independent film processing lab) will digitize film images for you. Additional record types such as visual fields, corneal topography, fluorescein angiograms, reports, and chart notes can also be stored in the database. This system provides a unique approach to digitizing, storing, retrieving, and viewing ophthalmic images. It is likely that more vendors will provide similar web-based ophthalmic imaging services in the future. You can find more information on OcuNet at www.ocunet.com.

Other methods of getting images into the computer include e-mail, web sites, and CDs. You can receive images from colleagues by e-mail or from web sites dedicated to image-hosting services. Web-based picture services enable users to upload images to a web server. The link (URL) to the specific page of images, or "Photo Album," can then be e-mailed to intended recipients so that they can

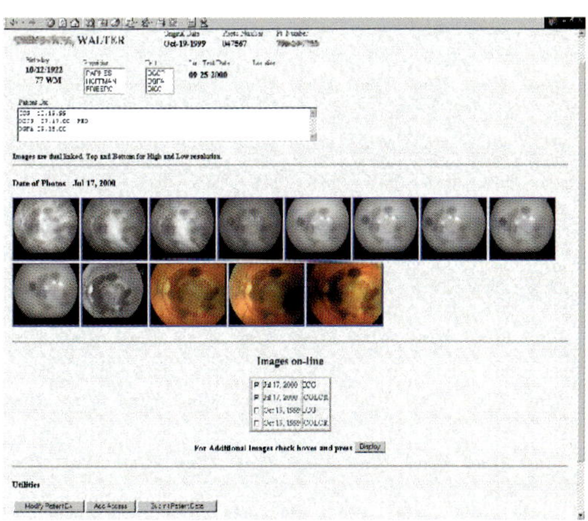

Figure 9–10 ○ A screen image from OcuNet's web-based image storage and retrieval software.

view or retrieve images. This service is often provided free or included as part of an Internet service contract. Some photo labs will process your film, then scan and upload the photos to a dedicated web site as part of their processing services. You (or those you share the photos with) can order high-quality prints directly from the hosting web site after your photos are uploaded. Some of these services provide password protection to restrict access to the image files. These services are meant for private, noncommercial use and are not practical for routine transfer of fundus images, but they do provide a way to share occasional photos and order high-quality prints. Dormant accounts are often deleted after a few months, and these services sometimes change their policies, merge, or go out of business, so do not consider this a stable, long-term image storage solution. Even though some services offer security features or password protection, do not include any confidential patient information if you share images in this way. Current examples of web sites that offer web-based picture services include the following:

www.nikonnet.com
www.ofoto.com
www.dotphoto.com
www.photo.epson.com
www.cartogra.com

It is also possible to download image files from web sites that permit copying. Always assume that all web content is copyrighted, and obtain permission before copying or using. Remember that the web is really just another method of publishing information, but instead of using paper, a network of computers is the medium of choice. You would never transcribe the words from a Hemingway novel or copy a painting by Van Gogh and sign your name to them. Think of electronic images in the same way. Some online images are protected with a digital watermark that is embedded in the image.

To copy an image from a web page, simply place the cursor on the image and then right-click (or click and hold with a one-button mouse). Choose "Save Image As" to save the image file to a folder on your computer. You can also copy the image and paste it into another application such as PowerPoint. Images or pages that are displayed by Adobe Acrobat Reader might not permit you to copy images, depending on the level of security that was selected when the file was created. Take a look at the following sites for some current examples of online ophthalmic image collections:

www.nyee.edu
(No copyright notice.)

www.nei.nih.gov/photo/index.htm
(Images are not copyrighted, but proper credit for use is requested.)

www.onjoph.com
(Images have a copyright notice on them and may be protected from unauthorized publishing with a digital watermark.)

www.images.md
(Subscription service to a database of over 40,000 medical images from different collections, including ophthalmology.)

You may also be able to find educational image collections on CD-ROM. CD-ROM image collections are sometimes published as a companion to ophthalmic textbooks. Image collections are typically copyrighted and may have some restrictions for their use. The Fair Use Statute of the U.S. Copyright Act permits the noncommercial, educational use of copyrighted materials without permission in certain circumstances. When in doubt, assume that any published image (from a journal, textbook, web page, CD, etc.) is copyrighted, and obtain appropriate permission before copying. A few examples of ophthalmic CD-ROM image collections are the following:

Chong NHV, Downes SM, Freeman GM, et al.: Medical Retina CD-ROM. London: BMJ Books, 1999.
Gass DJ: Stereoscopic Atlas of Macular Diseases: Diagnosis and Treatment CD-ROM. St. Louis: Mosby, 1999.
Kanski JJ, Nischal K: Clinical Ophthalmology CD-ROM: A Test Yourself Atlas. Boston: Butterworth-Heinemann, 2001.
Montzka DP: Wills Eye Hospital Atlas of Clinical Ophthalmology CD-ROM, 2nd ed. Philadelphia: Lippincott, Williams & Wilkins, 2001.
Parrish RK: Bascom Palmer Atlas of Ophthalmology. Boston: Butterworth-Heinemann, 1999.
Yannuzzi LA, Guyer DR, Green WR: The Retina Atlas CD-ROM. St. Louis: Mosby, 1998.
Yanoff M, Duker JS: Ophthalmology CD-ROM. St. Louis: Mosby, 1999.

Image File Management

Once you are successful at getting images into the computer, you will need to organize your image files. As you accumulate large numbers of images, move files from your computer hard drive to alternative storage: either a network server or external storage media such as Zip Disks, CD-R, or DVD. Archiving image files in this manner will free up space for new images on your hard drive. If you capture images with a commercially produced digital fundus camera, it is a simple matter to archive and retrieve images with the database that is provided with your system.

If you scan frequently or routinely export direct-captured images for use in publications or PowerPoint presentations, you will need to find another way to manage your image files. For low-volume use, you can simply create a sub-directory of folders and store image files as you would word-processing documents or other computer files. It does not take very long to outgrow this approach, however, and you might find a need for an image-cataloging program. After all, the best retinal images in the world are useless if they cannot be located and retrieved.

Some image-editing programs such as Photoshop and JASC Paint Shop Pro provide a browser utility that will create thumbnail images of all image files within a folder and display them in a proof sheet format. There are a number of stand-alone programs that function in the same way. They are useful for browsing your image folders to visually search for images. Some of these cataloging programs allow you to assign keywords and annotate images to store relevant information with the image file (Fig. 9–11).

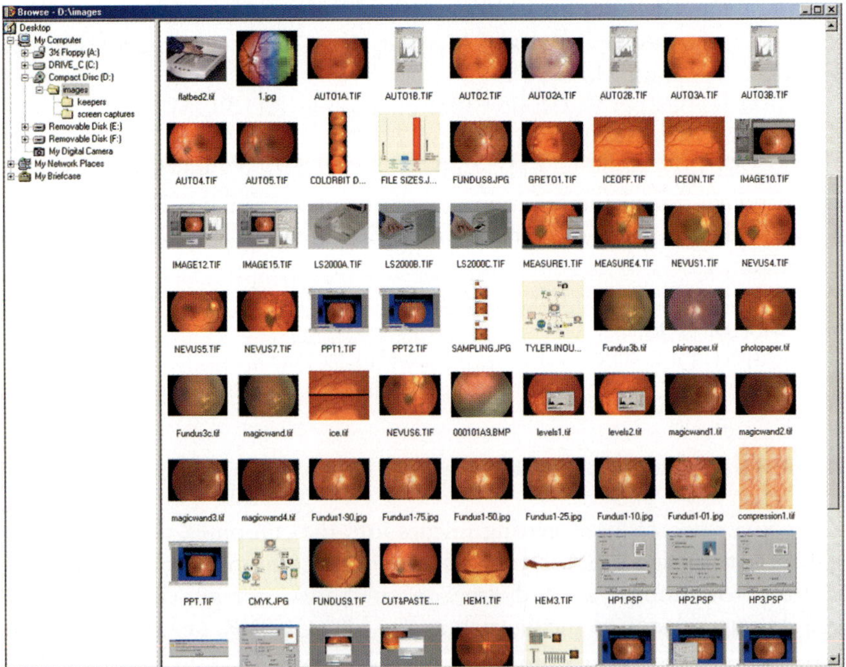

Figure 9–11 ○ Many imaging programs feature a Browse function that allows you to visually search image folders to easily locate and retrieve specific images. Your OS may also display thumbnail images of popular file formats.

More robust asset management programs offer greater flexibility in cataloging and retrieving digital files (sometimes termed *assets*) such as photos, video clips, and sound files. Extensis Portfolio, ACDSee, Canto Cumulus, and ThumbsPlus (Cerious Software) are popular asset management programs that will catalog image files through the use of predefined database fields along with searchable keywords and user-defined fields. These programs create thumbnails of images from most common image file formats and store them along with metadata in the database fields. The predefined fields are filled in automatically from information stored with the image file when it is loaded into the program. Once cataloged, image thumbnails can be browsed and images retrieved by searching keywords or fields. The programs do not actually store the image files them-selves but record a link to the file location for retrieval, whether they are stored on the hard drive, a server, or removable storage media. These programs are good image management solutions for those who store images outside the conventional image database of the commercial fundus imaging systems (Fig. 9–12).

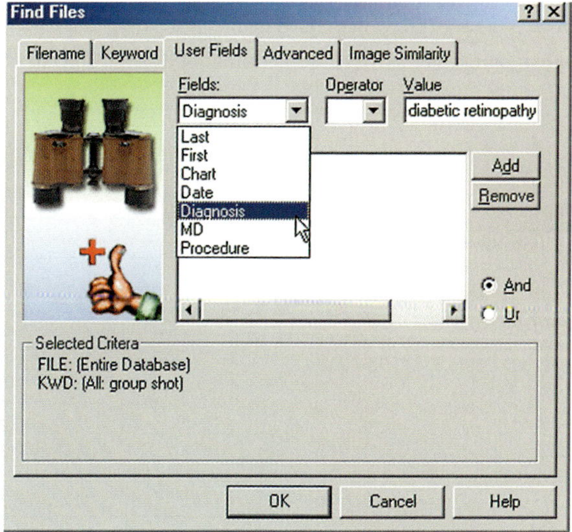

Figure 9–12 ○ Use asset management programs to visually browse thumbnail images in folders on your hard drive and removable storage media. You can also annotate the images, assign keywords, and define database fields to facilitate image retrieval. The Find Files dialog box in ThumbsPlus allows you to query the image database. In this example, the user has defined database fields for patient name, diagnosis, date, ordering physician, and procedure. The program will retrieve thumbnails of all images that meet the search criteria.

Reference

1. Scott JR: An affordable alternative to the high cost of digital fundus photography. J Ophthalmol Photog 2002;24:55.

Resources

Books and Articles

Blatner D, Roth S, Fleishman G: Real World Scanning and Halftones: The Definitive Guide to Scanning and Halftones from the Desktop, 2nd Edition. Berkeley: Peachpit Press, 1998.

Fulton W: A Few Scanning Tips, 2nd Edition. Self-published (www.scantips.com), 1999.

Mark G, Horvat L: Digital Imaging: Essential Skills. Boston: Butterworth-Heinemann, 2001.

Paynter H: What to look for in a desktop scanner. Photo Electronic Imaging 2000;43(4):38–43.

Rodney A: Correcting at the scan stage. Photo Electronic Imaging 1999; 42(1):18–26.

Rodney A: Step-by-step scanning. Photo Electronic Imaging 1998;41(6):40–47.

Saine PJ, Tyler ME: Ophthalmic Photography: Retinal Photography, Angiography, and Electronic Imaging, 2nd Edition. Boston: Butterworth-Heinemann, 2002.

Tally T: Avoiding the Scanning Blues: A Desktop Scanning Primer. Upper Saddle River: Prentice Hall PTR, 2000.

Web Sites

www.imaging-resource.com
www.kodak.com/US/en/digital/dlc/index.jhtml
www.scanhelp.com
www.scantips.com
www.shortcourses.com

Chapter 10

Digital Image Processing and Output

A major advantage of digital imaging is the ability to conveniently enhance or adjust your photos through image processing and easily share them in electronic and print form. This chapter describes the basic tenets of image processing as well as the secrets to high-quality printouts.

Ideally, all digital photographs would be perfect from the moment of capture, but in reality, most will benefit from image enhancement before being displayed or printed. The software that is supplied with commercial digital fundus imaging systems will allow you to adjust brightness, contrast, and sharpness for viewing and printing. For clinical diagnosis and printing, these basic tools are usually all that are necessary.

There may be times when you need to move beyond these basic tools to incorporate your fundus images into publications and presentations. A number of computer programs can help you make use of your digital fundus photographs by combining text, photos, and graphics (Table 10–1). There are, of course, additional software options. This listing contains software programs that we have found to be reliable and robust. In choosing software, the first step is always to determine your goal. What do you want to accomplish? To enhance your photographs, look for image-editing programs. If you want to use images in a presentation, look for presentation programs. For creating printed material and brochures, examine desktop publishing software.

Image-Editing Programs

Use an image-editing program for any image enhancement beyond the basic tools provided with your digital imaging system or scanning software. An image-editing program supplies a broad range of enhancement tools that allow you to

Table 10–1
Useful Programs and Their Features

Goal: Create or edit image files. Add vector labels to images.
Software Type Required: Image editing
Recommended Programs: Adobe Photoshop or Photoshop Elements, JASC Paint shop Pro
Features: Extensive image enhancements and correction, layers, channels, filters
File type: Bitmap images: *.bmp, *.tif, *.jpg, *.gif

Goal: Combine text and images for presentation
Software Type Required: Presentation Graphics
Recommended Programs: Microsoft PowerPoint
Features: Simple animation and low-resolution movies. Scientific poster layout is possible.
File type: Combination of bitmap and vector graphics: *.ppt, *.pps

Goal: Create or edit graphics. Modify (bends, twists, etc) text
Software Type Required: Drawing
Recommended Programs: Adobe Illustrator, Macromedia Freehand
Features: Graphics creation, drawing, illustrations, text composition. Layouts and basic image placement possible. Precise color control.
File type: Line art, vector graphics: *.eps
Output: Printer and prepress files

Goal: Simple combination of mostly text with some graphics
Software Type Required: Word-processing
Recommended Programs: Microsoft Word
Features: Text entry, simple image insertion
File type: Text document: *.doc, *.rtf, *.txt

Goal: Combine text and images for commercially printed projects, high-quality self-published material
Software Type Required: Desktop publishing
Recommended Programs: Adobe PageMaker, Adobe InDesign, QuarkXPress
Features: Layout and text design. Precise image placement and color control. Limited image resizing (+/–20%). Advanced publishing features and scientific poster layout.
File type: Page layout files with linked image files

Goal: Combine text and images for the web
Software Type Required: Web page design
Recommended Programs: Adobe GoLive, Macromedia DreamWeaver
Features: Web pages with linked URLs, web animation
File type: HTML files with linked image, data, or *.pdf files

Goal: Combine text and images for electronic distribution
Software Type Required: Electronic publishing
Recommended Programs: Adobe Acrobat
Features: File-formatting program that produces documents that will look the same on any operating system or with any program that can view or print a *.pdf file.
File type: Portable document files: *.pdf

adjust the quality of your images and prepare them for output. Think of an image-editing program as your "digital darkroom" (Fig. 10–1). It will enable you to maximize the quality of your fundus images and maybe even have some fun while doing it. Even if you have no darkroom experience, it does not take very long to learn the basics of image enhancement and output. Once you have mastered a few basics, the creative possibilities are endless.

But before you enter the digital darkroom and unleash your creativity, we should take a brief look at ethics and image enhancement. In most instances, we are taking retinal images for documentation or diagnosis, images that will be part of a patient's medical record. As medical professionals, we need to be keenly aware of how image-processing techniques can alter the diagnostic information

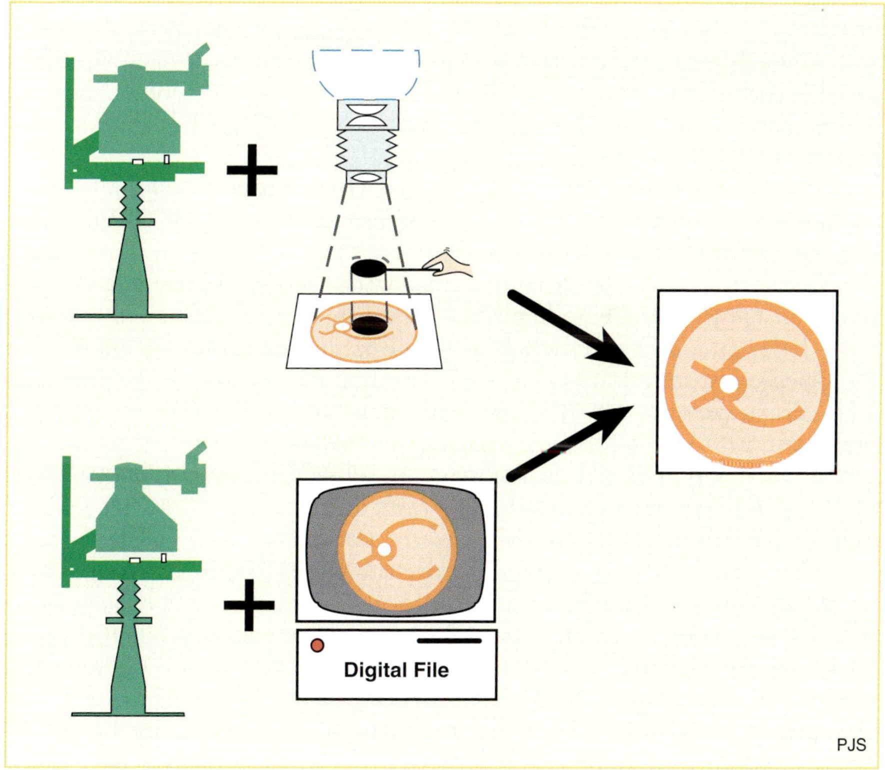

Figure 10–1 ○ Digital image enhancement techniques have replaced the traditional photographic darkroom for many fundus-imaging tasks. The "digital darkroom" provides a number of tools that allow you to easily adjust contrast, brightness, and color balance; remove artifacts; and create new illustrations by combining elements from multiple image sources. Many of these enhancements would be difficult or impractical in a traditional darkroom.

in a photograph. Enhancing diagnostic features through image processing is acceptable in the clinical environment. There is, however, a danger of overenhancement to the point of altering that diagnostic information. We have a responsibility to preserve the scientific integrity of our clinical images by judicious use of enhancement techniques and saving the original patient files in an unaltered form. When we begin to add or subtract diagnostic information through image processing, we will have crossed the line from photodocumentation to photo-illustration. This is acceptable only if it is clear that the resulting image is no longer a valid part of a patient's medical record. Keep this important distinction in mind when employing any image-processing techniques. If you decide to alter the images, you will need to understand the basic image-editing concepts that follow.

Adobe Photoshop is the industry standard for professional, high-end image editing. It provides a broad and powerful collection of imaging tools and is the program of choice for graphic designers and imaging professionals. It also comes with a high price tag and a steep learning curve. If you plan to do a lot of prepress image preparation or share your work with other imaging professionals, then you will probably want to use Photoshop. Corel PHOTO-PAINT is another well-known professional image-editing program.

If you are not quite ready to make the financial and educational commitment to Photoshop, programs such as Adobe Photoshop Elements, JASC Paint Shop Pro, and Ulead PhotoImpact are less expensive alternatives that are also easier to use. These lower-priced photo editors are powerful and flexible enough for most fundus imaging needs. Photoshop Elements is a "prosumer" offering from Adobe that is based on some of the core elements and features of Photoshop but without the expense and steep learning curve. Paint Shop Pro is a popular professional-level editing program for Windows with many of the tools found in higher priced competitors. Ophthalmic Imaging Systems includes this program as the default photo editor within their WinStation software for times when you want to go beyond the standard enhancement tools they provide. Of the full-featured programs, PhotoImpact may be the easiest to learn and use. Its feature set includes a number of tools that are specifically dedicated to preparing images for the web.

Many digital cameras and scanners provide a consumer-level image-editing program as part of a software bundle. Bundled image-editing programs vary in quality and feature sets. They may or may not provide you with the tools you need. MGI PhotoSuite, Adobe PhotoDeluxe, and Microsoft Picture It! are examples of basic image-editing programs that typically emphasize a graphics-based interface with automatic enhancement tools and templates for creating cards, calendars, and the like. They are great for producing holiday cards from retinal images and eliminating red-eye in your family photos, but they would likely be inadequate for most medical imaging needs. Besides, why would anyone want to ruin a perfectly good photograph by removing the fundus reflex with a red-eye removal tool?

If you are able to maximize image quality at capture, most fundus images will require only minor enhancement. Even though you might not need all of the sophisticated editing tools of the high-end editing programs, they usually do a better job of sizing, scaling, and preparing images for output. Digital fundus camera systems are typically optimized by the manufacturer for proper contrast and color balance and usually will not need additional correction. If you acquire photographs with a scanner, follow the instructions for optimizing scan quality (in Chapter 9) to minimize the amount of postscan processing needed for these images. Some images, however, will benefit from more extensive image enhancement, especially those that are captured under less than ideal circumstances (media opacities, small pupil, unwanted reflexes from IOLs, etc).

The following sections discuss common image-editing tools that you will find useful for fundus photography. All of the major image-editing applications will have these or similar tools. This is not meant to be a tutorial for each tool; it is simply a brief introduction to what these commands do and some tips for use.

Useful Commands, Tools, and Features

Save

The act of saving computer files is such a fundamental part of computer technique that you might wonder why it is included in this list. There are a few very important reasons. One of the first rules of image editing is to make a copy of the original image and make all editing changes to the copy. Having a master copy is useful if you need to revert back to the original if a file is damaged during editing. The peace of mind that comes with knowing that you have an archived master copy of the image will free you to experiment and try different editing techniques.

"Save early, save often" is the mantra of many imaging professionals. You should save your image after any major editing change or after every few minor changes. Image processing can put a significant strain on your computer's system resources, and failures can occur when least expected. Save your changes frequently to protect yourself from having to start the editing process from scratch if a failure occurs.

Save As

The *Save As* command is useful at the beginning and end of the editing process. If your original image is acquired in a lossy format (JPEG), you will want to save it in a lossless format while editing. If you edit and save changes frequently, a JPEG image will lose quality each time you save and reopen in this format. After you open a JPEG file for editing, save it as a TIFF or other lossless file format.

The best choice for saving an image in process is probably the format that is native to your image editor (for example, Photoshop's *.psd format), which allows you to take advantage of the layers editing feature.

The *Save As* command is often used again at the completion of the editing process to convert the image to JPEG, TIFF, or another universal format that is appropriate for display or distribution. (See the descriptions of file formats in Chapter 8.)

Undo/Redo

You will use this command often. As the name implies, it allows you to undo an action that has an unintended effect or degrades the image. After undoing an action, if you decide that it looked better after all, simply use the *Redo* command to restore the changes. Multiple levels of undo are available in some programs. In Photoshop, the History pallet acts as the multiple undo command.

Layers

Many image-editing programs support this feature. It is useful for combining elements from multiple raster (bitmapped) images or adding vector graphics, text, or geometric shapes such as arrows in a separate layer (Fig. 10–2). When you save in a format that does not support this feature (TIFF, JPEG, or GIF), all layers are merged together and can no longer be edited separately. Vector graphics or text may suffer a loss in quality when converted to a merged bitmap, so you might want to keep a file copy in the editor's native file format.

Selection Tools

Selection tools designate a portion of an image for editing. The selected area is usually surrounded by a blinking outline called a *Marquee*. If you have a fundus image that is unevenly exposed, you can use one of the selection tools to select a specific area for enhancement or brightening without affecting the remainder of the image (Fig. 10–3). Typical selection tools include a rectangle or other geometric shape that can be dragged over the desired area, a *Lasso* or freehand drawing tool and something known as a *Magic Wand*. The Lasso tool may have an option that utilizes edge detection to simplify drawing a selection outline along an edge. To use this option, either trace or click-and-drag along a pixel edge, and the tool detects the exact border for you. The Magic Wand selects an area by identifying pixels of similar brightness or color. To use this tool, point-and-click on an area, and the Magic Wand automatically selects pixels of similar tone and color. You can adjust the sensitivity threshold of this tool to control how much area it selects. Feather the selected area to blend smoothly.

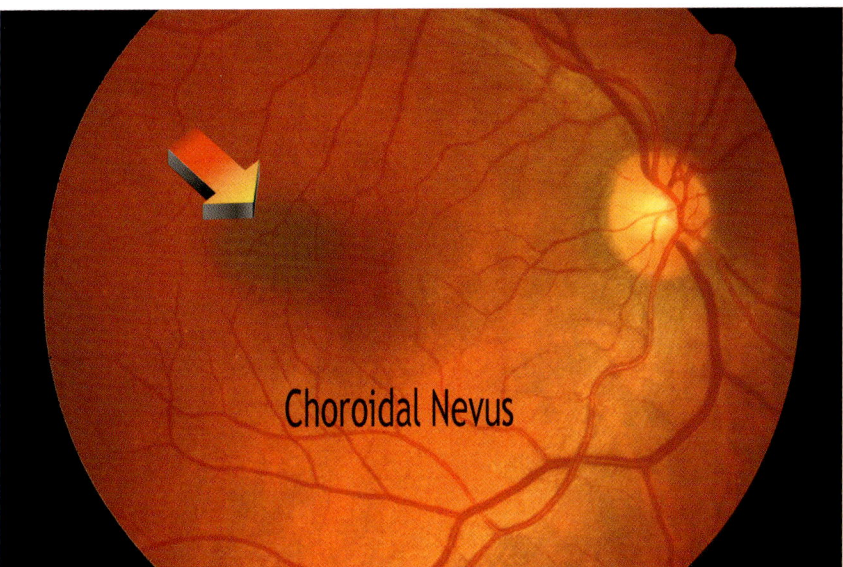

Figure 10–2 ◯ A fundus photograph with text and a vector arrow added in a separate layer. The vector graphic can be moved, scaled, rotated, and edited for color and fill properties until the vector and bitmap layers are merged and saved in a universal file format that does not support separate layers (e.g., TIFF, JPEG).

Crop

This tool is not usually necessary in fundus photography, since the magnification of the image is generally set at capture. The most common use of this tool is to crop images scanned from 35-mm film to change the aspect ratio for screen display or to display just a portion of the image. The aspect ratio of 35-mm film is 3:2. Cropping some of the black mask from the sides of a fundus image can reduce the width to achieve a screen aspect ratio of 4:3. Cropping is preferable to resampling when making a change in aspect ratio.

Rotate

Use this tool to correct images that were scanned at a slight angle. Some cropping is necessary after rotating at settings other than 90 or 180 degrees.

Brightness/Contrast

This is a simple, useful tool with an intuitive interface that uses a set of sliders to increase or decrease brightness and contrast. A common use would be to increase

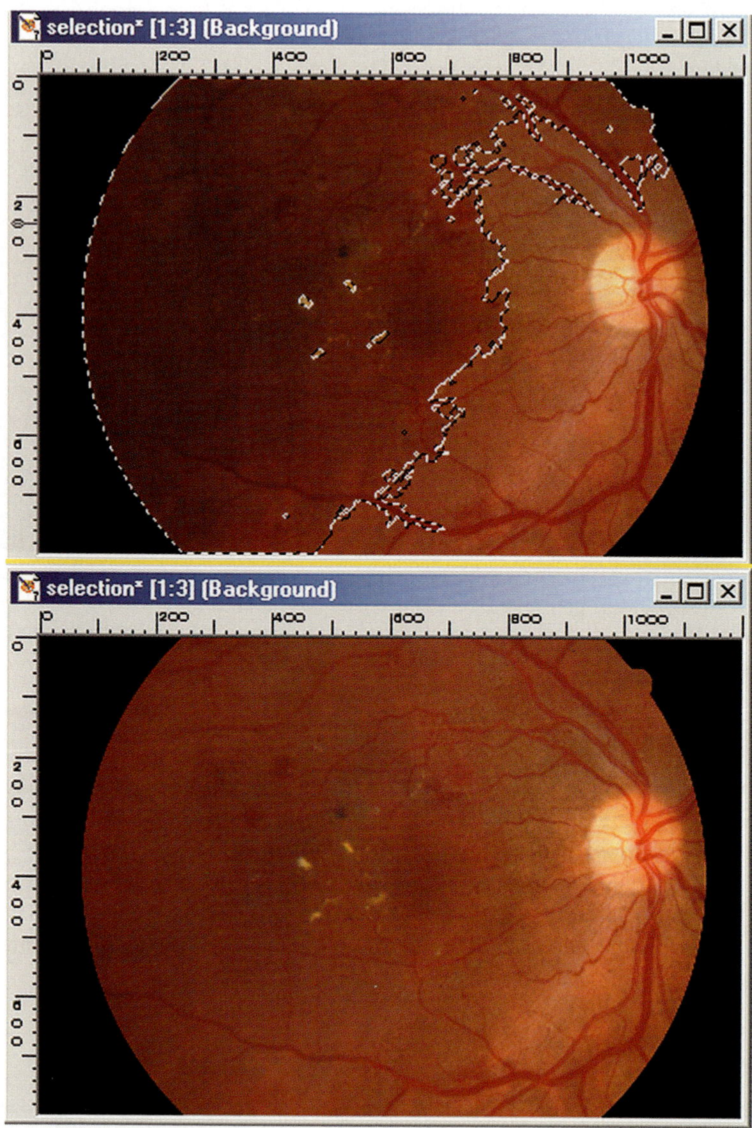

Figure 10–3 ○ Inadequate pupillary dilation often causes uneven illumination and exposure. *Top,* The Magic Wand selection tool was used to select the underexposed area in this photograph of a patient who was not maximally dilated. The threshold of the tool was adjusted until it selected only the dark area. *Bottom,* The corrected image shows an increase in brightness and contrast in the previously selected area.

contrast in fundus images that exhibit reduced contrast from media opacities such as cataracts.

Levels (Histogram)

This tool is just like the one you use to maximize tonal values prior to scanning. It offers more control than the simple sliders of the *Brightness/Contrast* tool, adjusting the dark, light, and midtone values separately. The histogram provides a graphic representation of the distribution of pixels in an image based on their brightness. Use the histogram to help you determine what tonal corrections may be appropriate for your image. (See the section entitled "Scanning Techniques" in Chapter 9 for a description of histogram use.)

Curves

This is a more advanced tool for adjusting brightness, contrast, and color rendition. Instead of being limited to the single adjustment parameter of the Brightness/Contrast tool or the three control points found in *Levels*, with *Curves* you can choose multiple, tonal areas for adjustment. Changes can be made to each color channel separately.

Color Balance

This is another intuitive interface that uses sliders to adjust the color balance of your images by increasing or decreasing the amount of each color channel. Make your color balance changes after adjusting brightness and contrast. Retinal images usually do not need much color correction, since fundus camera flash illumination provides consistent color rendition. Color correction is more commonly used with scanned slide duplicates or photographic prints with color shifts.

Grayscale

This easy-to-use command converts a color image to a continuous-tone black-and-white image. It can be used in preparing photographs for publications that require grayscale images (Fig. 10–4). Selecting the green channel before making a grayscale conversion will darken the red blood vessels and increase overall contrast, producing an image similar to a green filter fundus photograph with black-and-white film.

Clone

This is a very useful select-and-copy tool that will let you copy part of an image to another location. It is helpful for retouching artifacts. Cloning between images

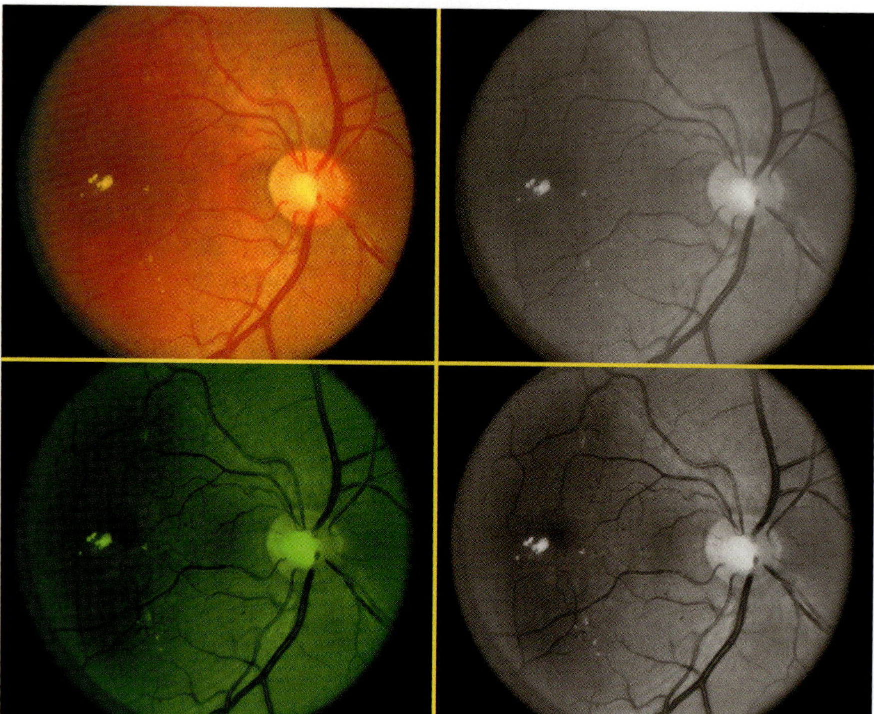

Figure 10–4 ○ Use the *Grayscale* command to remove color from an image. It will convert the image to an 8-bit grayscale image by replacing colors with a gray value of equal luminance. *Upper left,* Full-color, 24-bit image. *Upper right,* Grayscale conversion. *Lower left,* Color image placed in the green channel to approximate the view through a monochromatic green, "red-free" filter. *Lower right,* Grayscale conversion of the green image darkens the blood vessels and increases overall contrast.

will enable you to combine elements of both. You could, for example, copy a hemorrhage, lesion, or other diagnostic feature from one fundus photo and paint it into another to create an illustration for educational purposes (Fig. 10–5). However, such an altered image should not be included in a patient's medical record.

Dust and Scratches

This image-processing filter is helpful in removing noise, dust, and scratch artifacts from scanned originals but may reduce image sharpness.

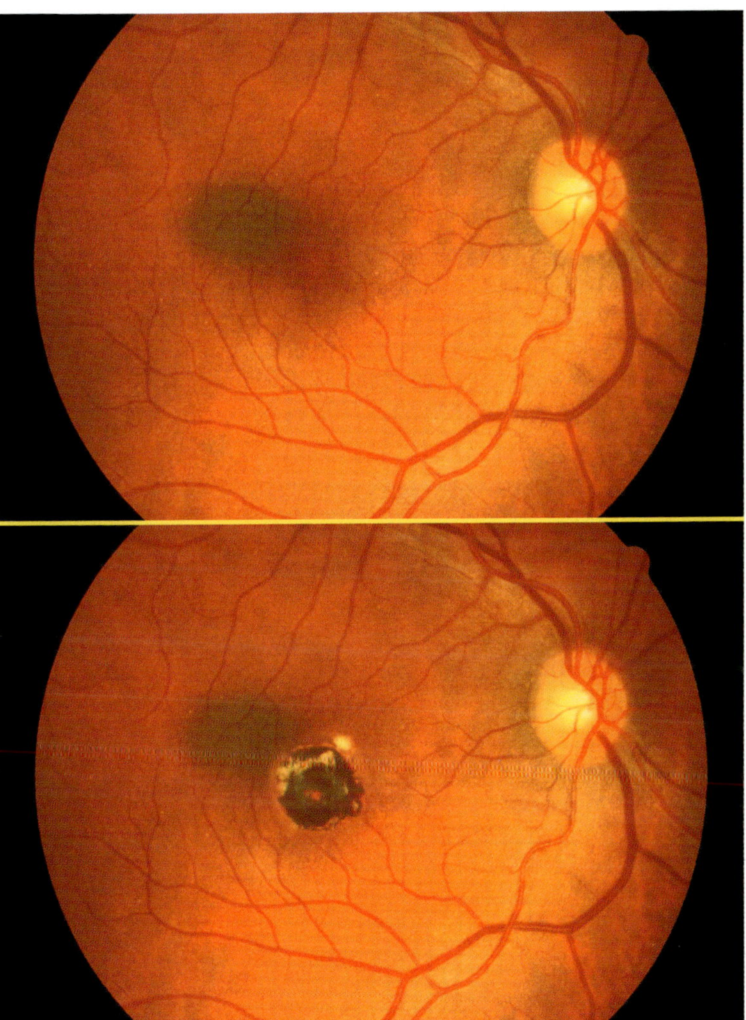

Figure 10–5 ○ *Top*, Fundus image of a choroidal nevus as captured by the fundus camera. *Bottom*, A clone tool was used to insert a pigmented scar copied from a different photo to create a new image. This new image may be useful for illustration purposes but is no longer a valid part of a patient's medical record. A more common use of this tool is to retouch dust spots or other artifacts by cloning pixels from an adjacent area of the same image.

Moiré Pattern Removal

The *Moiré Removal* filter works like the tool found in most scanner drivers to remove the unwanted dot patterns that often appear in scans of halftone printed originals. (See Fig. 9–8 in the previous chapter.)

Image Size/Resize

The most efficient way to deal with image file sizes is to scan or acquire the original image at the desired output resolution. If you are unable to size the image during capture, the *Image Size* command is used for sizing and scaling images for output. The dialog box that appears for this command will allow you to size an image on the basis of pixel dimensions, print size, and, in some programs, percentage of original.

Photoshop's *Image Size* dialog box has two check boxes that are very important (Fig. 10–6). The first one, *Constrain Proportions*, should usually remain checked. This maintains the image aspect ratio. (Paint Shop Pro calls this check box

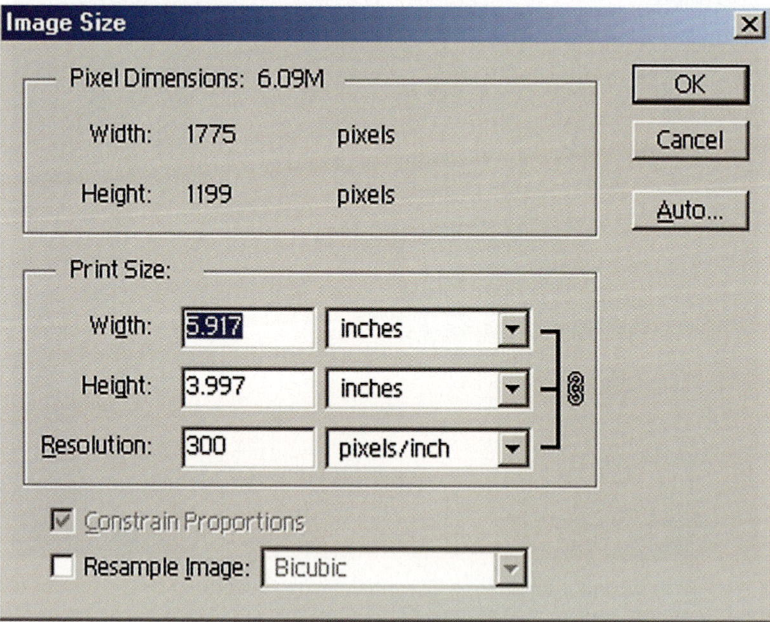

Figure 10–6 ○ The Photoshop Image Size dialog box displays the pixel dimensions of the image. Use this box to scale your image to the appropriate print size using percent, inches, centimeters, points, or picas. To maintain the image aspect ratio, leave the Constrain Proportions box checked. Do not check the Resample Image box unless you want to invent or discard pixels. In most cases, the Bicubic algorithm will give you the best result when resampling.

Maintain aspect ratio.) If this box is unchecked, resampling may use two different scales between the two image axes, causing the picture to look stretched in one direction. Cropping is usually the best way to change the aspect ratio.

The second check box is called *Resample Image.* If you want to scale an image to a specific output size, leave this box unchecked. Scaling is preferable to resampling when sizing an image, because it does not affect the pixel count. It simply specifies the physical dimensions for printing. In scaling, the dialog box can act as a "scaling calculator." Resampling changes image size by inventing or discarding pixels. When resampling is necessary, you usually want to use the *Bicubic* sampling algorithm (if your image-editing program gives you a choice). Sharpening is often helpful after resampling an image. For more information on resizing images, see the discussion on resolution and resizing in Chapter 8.

Sharpen (Sharpen More, Unsharp Mask)

Most programs will give you a choice of different commands to increase apparent image sharpness. *Sharpen* filters work by identifying pixel transitions, defining edges, and then increasing the contrast between adjacent pixels. *Sharpen* and *Sharpen More* are automatic sharpening filters that often work well. They can be applied multiple times, but oversharpening will create unwanted noise in the image. *Unsharp Mask* is a command that offers greater control over the sharpening effect (Fig. 10–7). You can adjust the parameters for amount, radius, and threshold. *Amount* controls the amount by which contrast is increased. A good starting point is 100–150%. *Radius* specifies the area surrounding the edge pixels. A higher number will define a larger area of pixels for sharpening. A setting of 1–2 is usually appropriate if the image has already been sized for final output. *Threshold* is the brightness difference between pixels that determines which pixels are identified as edge pixels. A setting of 0 will sharpen all pixels, which is usually too extreme for fundus images. Try a setting between 5 and 10. Do not be afraid to experiment with this tool; it can work wonders. Sharpening is usually the last enhancement that is applied before saving the final image.

Image Output

Image output is the final step in the digital imaging process. If you have captured your images at the appropriate size and resolution and then enhanced them for proper contrast, exposure, and color balance, the image is ready for display. Display can take a number of different forms. Reviewing direct-captured images on a computer monitor is the most common and obvious method of digital image output in fundus photography. After capturing images with a digital fundus camera, you can easily review them with a colleague or patient.

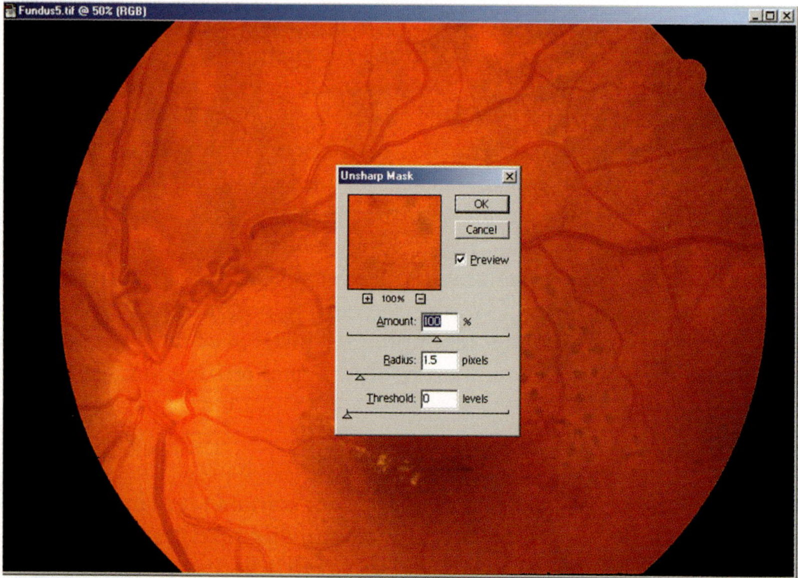

Figure 10–7 ○ The Unsharp Mask filter allows you to set controls for Amount, Radius, and Threshold. *Amount* relates to the strength of the filter. Start with 100 percent. *Radius* controls the number of pixels around an edge that are affected. Try a setting of 1. Increase this number for high-resolution images or images that will be printed. *Threshold* specifies the amount of contrast adjacent pixels must have before they are sharpened. A threshold of 0 means that all pixels are affected. For fundus images, start with a setting of 5. Increase this setting if the image appears "noisy." Low numbers are often appropriate for highly detailed images.

Computer networks will allow you to upload fundus photographs to remote computers or a server and display them on monitors in additional locations such as examination lanes or laser suites. This type of image distribution usually requires the same software package that is used by the capture system to access images through the patient database. Archive discs, usually CDs, can also be used to move images to different computers for display. Direct-capture systems are often configured with a dye-sublimation or high-quality inkjet printer to make prints for the patient's medical record, providing another image output medium.

Viewing in a software application different from the one that is used for capture may require exporting the images in a universal file format such as TIFF, PNG, or JPEG. Once an image has been exported, you lose the convenience of the patient database provided by the capture program, so consider naming the images files in a way that lets you identify them by patient name and capture date.

Converting some images to a universal file format will allow you to utilize them in other programs. Images can be inserted into word-processing or desktop publishing documents to produce referral letters, reports, informational brochures, or other printed publications. Presentation graphics programs such as Power-Point let you incorporate fundus images into educational lectures for onscreen display or output to a film recorder for 35-mm slides.

This is why we stress knowing the intended output medium and image resolution before scanning or scaling. File format, compression levels, image processing, resampling, scanner interpolation, printer interpolation, printer settings, and paper choice can all affect the final resolution of an image. Managing these factors during all phases of the imaging process will produce the best possible image output.

Printing Digital Images

Printers vary in their capabilities and image quality. Some printers work exclusively as photo printers, while others can handle a combination of text and graphics. The printer that is supplied with your digital system may be all that you need. You will be able to print directly from the image-capture software supplied with your system. If you need to choose a printer, review the following description of printer types to help you decide what will work best in your practice setting. Manufacturers employ a number of different printing technologies; the two most popular types for digital photography are inkjet and dye-sublimation printers.

Color inkjet printers have become quite popular for printing digital photographs. Relatively inexpensive and versatile, they are often the best choice for low-volume home or business use. Various types of paper or media can be used to print a mix of text, graphics, and photographs. You can vary the resolution of the inkjet printer according to your needs. For example, quick drafts can be made on plain paper with low dpi settings to conserve ink. Inkjet printers often exhibit dot gain, or bleeding of colors, because of the fibrous nature of paper. For output that approaches "photo quality," use high-quality coated papers. Coated papers absorb less ink than plain paper, resulting in sharper edges and more vibrant colors (Fig. 10–8). When inkjet printers are used properly, their photographic output can be impressive. Instructions for printing fundus photographs on an inkjet printer are given in the accompanying box, "Printing a Fundus Photo on an injet Printer."

Standard color inkjet printers use *CMYK* (cyan, magenta, yellow, and black) inks. Black ink is added to the three subtractive primary colors to improve overall contrast and increase shadow density. A print head moves back and forth across the paper, building up an image by depositing drops of ink through very

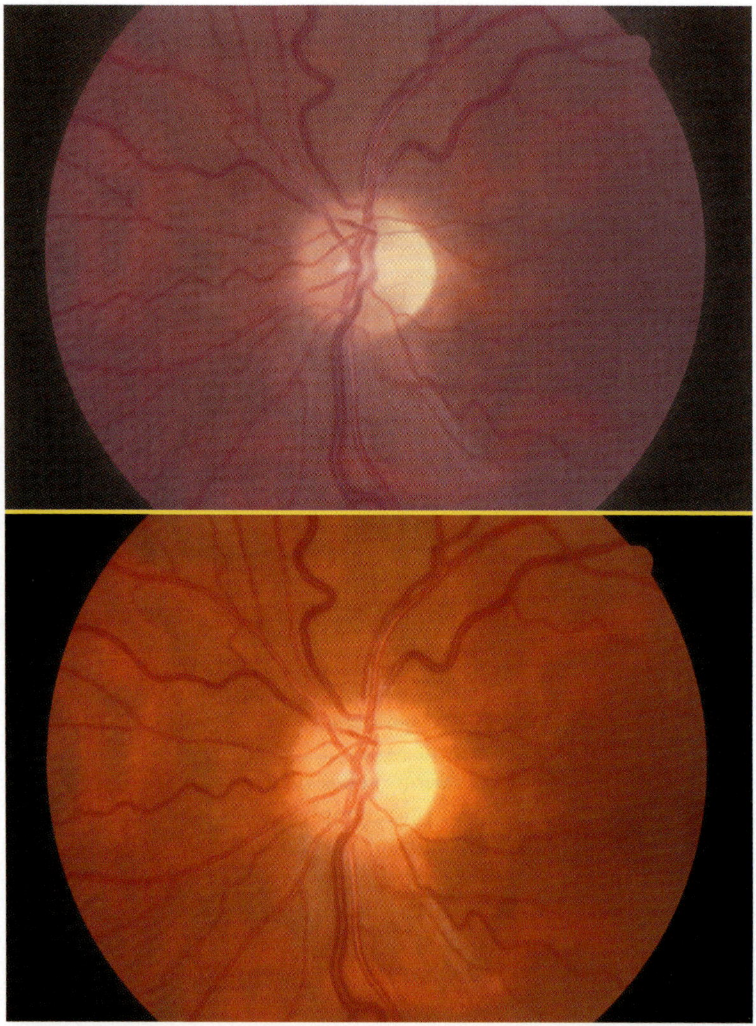

Figure 10–8 ○ Paper makes a difference in the quality of inkjet prints. Two versions of the same fundus image printed on two different paper types using an Epson 900 inkjet printer. *Top,* Image printed on plain paper using the highest quality settings. *Bottom,* Image printed on Epson Photo Quality Glossy Film using the same printer settings.

Printing a Fundus Photo on an Inkjet Printer

1. *Open the image file in the application you will be printing from.*
2. *Open* Page Setup *under the File menu to display general printing options. The appearance of the dialog box will vary with different programs, operating systems, and printers but will usually allow you to choose printer, paper size, paper source, orientation, scaling, and position on the page. You may also find options for printing gray-scale, negative, or CMYK separation images. Most likely, you will use the default color setting for fundus images.*
3. *Select the desired printer, paper size, and source.*
4. *Set the orientation to* Landscape *if you want the fundus photograph to fill the page. If you want to print more than one image on the page, you might want to use* Portrait *orientation. Printing in the portrait mode may be faster with certain inkjet printers.*
5. *If you have scaled or sized your image appropriately (and by this point in the book, we hope you have), leave the scaling at 100%.*
6. *Select the location of the image on the page. Some programs will center the image on the page unless you specify other margins. Some programs provide a* Center on page *check box.*
7. *Click* OK *to save these settings. You may also be able to access the page setup controls under* Properties *in the* Print *dialog box.*
8. *Select* Print *from the* File *menu to open the print dialog box. Different options will be available, depending on the printer brand and model.*
9. *Click on* Properties, *and select the paper or media type you want to use. This is probably THE most important step in printing on an inkjet printer. When you select the paper type, your printer will load automatic print settings optimized for that medium.*
10. *Select a print quality setting. Most Hewlett-Packard printers offer print settings of* Draft, Normal, *or* Best, *(Fig. 10–9) while Epson's basic settings are* Normal, Fine, *and* Photo. *Other brands will have similar choices. Click on the* Custom *Button and then the* Advanced *button in the Epson print dialog box to select a resolution setting in dpi. The advanced settings for different printer models may have controls for adjusting the color balance, brightness, or color management settings (Fig. 10–10). For photo-quality output on good paper, select the highest setting. If you are printing a mix of text and bitmapped photos, good results can be obtained by using inkjet paper and medium quality settings. Inkjet paper is a thin paper stock that is brighter and absorbs less ink than plain paper. Paper selection is the key to high-quality inkjet output.*
11. *Place the appropriate paper stock in the paper tray, making sure the coated side is facing in the correct direction. On some models, the printing surface needs to face up; on others, it must face down. Some papers use a watermark or corner notch to aid in proper orientation.*
12. *Select the number of copies to print, and click* OK.
13. *If you are printing at photo-quality settings (1200/1440 dpi), find something useful to do for the next several minutes. It would be a good time to answer your e-mail except that your computer will probably be too busy writing the print job to the printer.*

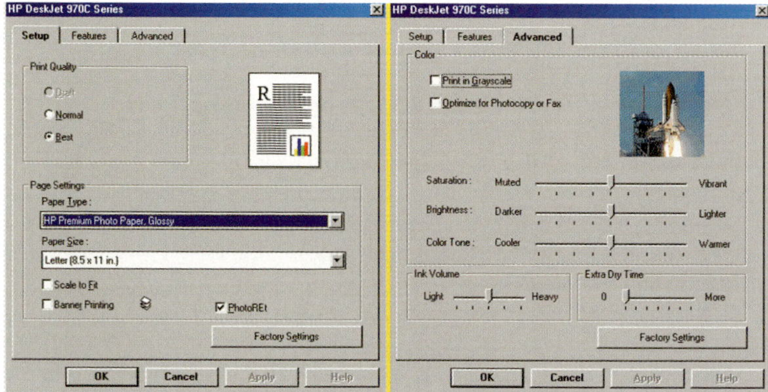

Figure 10–9 ○ The basic and advanced print dialog boxes for a Hewlett-Packard Deskjet 970c printer. The basic dialog box has settings for Print Quality and Paper Settings. Use the Advanced box to adjust print quality by moving the sliders for Saturation, Brightness, and Color Tone. It also provides adjustments for Ink Volume and Extra Dry Time.

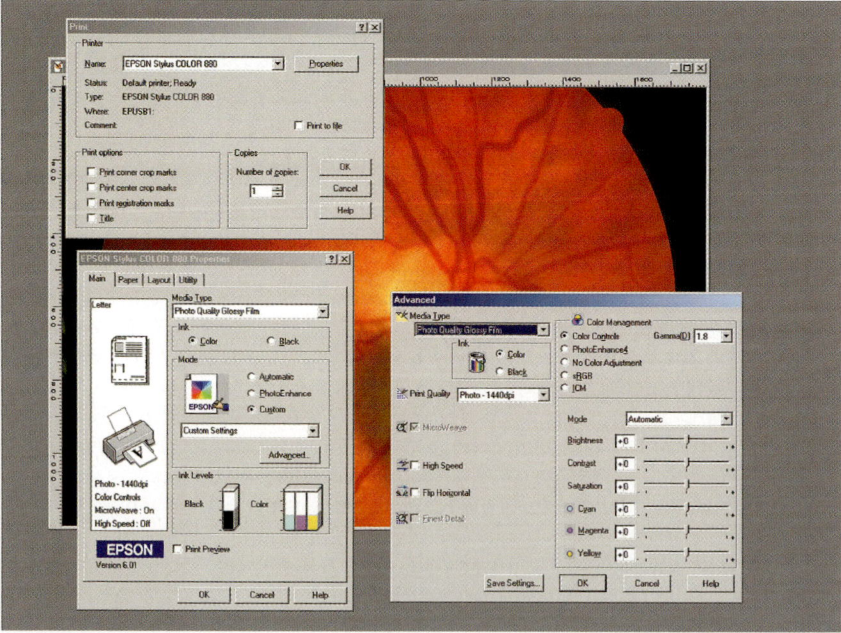

Figure 10–10 ○ Epson print dialog boxes. After selecting the desired printer and number of copies, click on Properties to set the paper type and quality settings. Automatic settings often work well, or you can select from a menu of automatic, custom, or color management settings in the Advanced dialog box. Use the Gamma control to adjust print output to more closely match monitor brightness.

small nozzles. The drops are blended by half-toning or dithering techniques to create the appearance of an extensive color palette. The driver software accepts RGB (red, green, blue) data, converts it to CMYK, and then determines the dot pattern and the amount of ink delivered to the page. Certain "photo-quality" printers use six ink colors, adding light cyan and light magenta to achieve better reproduction of subtle, continuous-tone subjects such as flesh tones.

The major disadvantages of inkjet printers are the slow speed and the expense of consumables, especially when you use the high quality settings necessary for printing photographs. Ink cartridges need to be changed often, and the special coated papers designed for photo printing are expensive. The flexibility in choosing different paper stock is an advantage.

The light-duty nature of most desktop inkjet printers is a disadvantage for high-volume work settings. Small ink cartridges need to be changed often, and the jets can easily clog. New business inkjet models, such as the HP 2200 series, may improve high-volume performance by utilizing long-life replaceable print heads, large separate ink cartridges, and a large sturdy paper tray.

When preparing images for inkjet printing, it is important to differentiate between the printer dpi and the image dpi (or, more accurately, the image ppi) that we use to describe the number of pixels in an image. Inkjet printer dpi refers to the number of ink droplets a printer can deliver to the page. It takes a number of inkjet dots or droplets to create one pixel. Consequently, inkjet printer dpi numbers are often significantly higher than the numbers we use to express pixel resolution. A common rule of thumb is to scale the image to final size at one-third of the dpi setting used on the printer, up to a maximum of 300 ppi. For an inkjet printer set at 720 dpi, an image sized at 240 ppi would be appropriate. Use the one-third rule as a starting point, but you might still end up with more pixel resolution than necessary for your printer. Some printers may have a "sweet spot," or an image resolution that the printer drivers are most comfortable interpolating. You should experiment with different print resolution settings on your inkjet printer to find out what resolution it "prefers." Recommendations for the appropriate image ppi settings may also vary by manufacturer. When in doubt, check the owner's manual for your printer or contact the manufacturer's tech-support service for a recommendation.

Dye sublimation, or "dye-sub," printers are continuous-tone color printers designed specifically for creating high-quality graphic arts and photographic output. Dye-sub printers produce images by transferring dyes from a plastic film or ribbon containing page-sized panels of cyan, magenta, and yellow dyes. A thermal print head, capable of precise temperature variations, moves across the transfer ribbon, vaporizing the dye in proportion to the amount of heat used. The dye then diffuses onto the paper surface. Each dye layer is transferred separately. This process precisely controls the amount of dye, resulting in output that is very close to true photographic quality.

Print speeds are quite slow, as the printer makes four passes over the same sheet of paper to deliver three color layers and a protective coating. Dye-sub printers do a poor job of reproducing text. Unlike color laser or inkjet printers, dye-sub printers can print only on paper stock that is specifically designed for this printing method. The combined cost of the printing ribbon and special paper stock make the cost of consumables quite high for dye-sub printing. Letter-sized prints cost about $3 per page. If photographic quality is more important than text, cost, or speed, then dye-sub printers are the best choice.

Unlike inkjet printers, the output dpi (dots per inch) of dye-sub printers can be equated with image ppi (pixels per inch). A dye-sub printer with an output resolution of 300 dpi will print a 300-ppi image with a one-for-one dot-to-pixel ratio. This makes the process of scanning or scaling to an appropriate resolution quite simple.

Thermo-autochrome print technology is different from other color printing methods. Instead of using ribbons or ink cartridges to transfer dyes, heat-sensitive CMY color pigments are incorporated within the paper stock. Each color layer is sensitive to a different temperature. It is somewhat analogous to the photographic process except that heat rather than light is used to activate each dye layer. The print stock has the look and feel of photographic paper.

Color laser printers are known for producing sharp text and graphics but are also capable of rendering near-photographic image quality. You can use different paper stock, including plain paper, but images will look best on paper that is designed for photo output. Laser printers are faster than inkjets, and although the initial cost is high, the consumable costs are usually lower than the cost of inkjet supplies. Laser printers are a good choice for printing a variety of text and graphics in high-volume settings, but their photographic output is not as good as that of other color printing technologies.

Fujifilm Pictrography printers utilize thermal development and dye-transfer technology to produce high-quality, continuous-tone color prints. This process combines a light-sensitive silver-halide material with laser diode exposure to create photographic prints in a variety of paper sizes without conventional photographic chemistry. You can choose from analog resolution settings of 133, 200, 267, 320,or 400 ppi.

Presentation Graphics

Use presentation graphics programs to incorporate photographic images into lectures and slide shows. Microsoft PowerPoint is the most commonly used presentation program, but programs such as Harvard Graphics and Corel Freelance are similar. While all of these programs will allow to you to print to a film recorder to produce 35-mm slides, the current trend is to present lectures electronically on a monitor or LCD computer projector. Just five years ago, virtually all lectures presented at the Ophthalmic Photographers' Society Annual Education Program used traditional 35-mm slides. By 2002, over 80% of the lectures were presented electronically. You can easily update lecture content or adjust to different audiences using electronic presentation. Another advantage is the ability to use the same fundus image (or multiple images) in multiple lectures.

The popularity of electronic presentation does not mean that 35-mm slides and 2-by-2 slide projectors are obsolete. Many institutions have huge archives of high-quality 35-mm educational fundus images. Rather than going to the expense and trouble of scanning these images for PowerPoint presentations, it is sometimes more appropriate to project the originals. Fundus images lend themselves to side-by-side display to show both eyes together. You can also do this by combining two images on a single slide in PowerPoint, but the magnification and image quality will not be as good as they are in side-by-side 35-mm projection. Some presenters also feel more secure with a traditional slide projector because, as with any high-tech process, there can be technical glitches. For major electronic presentations some presenters also keep 35-mm slides as a backup in case of problems with the computer or video projector. Whichever type of output you use, presentation software can enhance the educational content of your lectures by combining text and graphics with fundus images.

The first step in starting a PowerPoint presentation is to select the Page Setup for the intended display format (Fig. 10–11). The most commonly used formats are *On-screen Show* and *35mm Slides*. The image aspect ratio changes when you change the page setup, so you want to specify this *before* importing bitmapped images. If you do not do this, the horizontal image dimension will be compressed or stretched, distorting the image when you reset the aspect ratio.

Inserting images into PowerPoint is quite simple, but once again, the original should be sized appropriately (Table 10–2). PowerPoint presentations that contain numerous bitmapped images will result in large files that may slow performance. Sizing your image files before inserting them will result in smaller, more efficient PowerPoint files. Check the resolution of the monitor or LCD projector you will be using, and work backwards from this setting to determine the appropriate resolution and color-depth settings for your images. You can easily access these settings on a PC monitor by right-clicking on the desktop and then looking under *Properties*. If your monitor is set to display True Color (24 or 32 bit) at XGA resolution (1024 × 768), then use pixel dimensions of 1024 × 768 to fill the frame of a PowerPoint slide. You can also scan to a percentage of full pixel resolution to import an image at less than full-frame size. Scaling at 50–60% of the full-frame size will allow you to insert a fundus image into a frame with room for a text heading or description.

Another common method of setting resolution is to size the image to 7.5 × 10 inches at 72–100 ppi. This is the page layout size for *On-screen Show* in

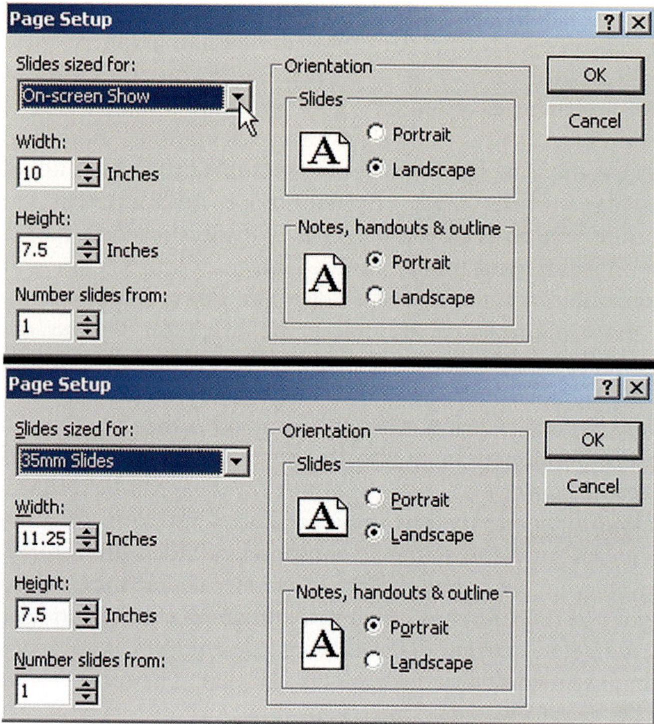

Figure 10–11 ○ Use PowerPoint's Page Setup to specify intended output size and aspect ratio before importing images into your presentation. Changing from *On-screen Show* to *35mm Slides* increases the page width and aspect ratio.

Table 10–2
How to Insert an Image into a PowerPoint Slide

1. Display the slide you want to import the image to.
2. Click on the *Insert* menu.
3. Select *Picture* and then *From File. . . .*
4. Browse to the folder that contains the image you want to insert.
5. Highlight the desired picture file.
6. To embed the image into PowerPoint, click *Insert*.
7. To link an image file instead of embedding it, click the arrow next to *Insert* to activate the drop-down menu. Select *Link to File*.
8. The image will appear centered within the slide frame.

PowerPoint. You can always scale the image within PowerPoint to fine-tune the size after inserting, but the idea is to get it close from the start. If intended output is to a film recorder, consider increasing the file resolution. Scan or size to the output resolution of the film recorder. Good results can also be obtained by scanning at 150 ppi at the page size of 7.5 × 11.25 to produce 35-mm slide images. If you change the page setup after images have been inserted, it will alter the aspect ratio of the inserted images. To reset the image to its original size and aspect ratio, select the *Size* tab in the *Format Picture* dialog box, unlock the aspect ratio, and then set the height and width scale to the original percentages. You will need to do this for every image in the presentation, so it is more efficient to set the page size correctly before importing image files (Fig. 10–12).

Images can be inserted from existing image files or direct from a scanner or digital camera. You can also copy and paste from another application. For best

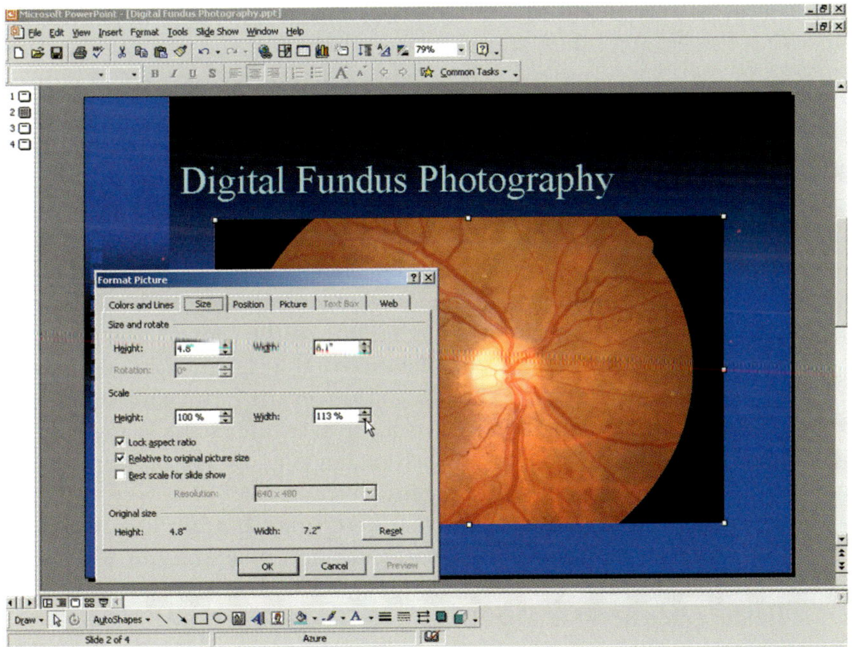

Figure 10–12 ○ If you change the page setup of a presentation containing photographs, you might change the image aspect ratio. To reset the aspect ratio, open the Format Picture box and select the Size tab. In this example the Page Setup was changed from On-screen show to 35mm Slides. Note that the image is stretched on its horizontal axis and the size scale shows an image width of 113%. To change this, deselect the Lock aspect ratio checkbox and set the width to 100%. You will need to do this for every image in a presentation if you change the initial page setup selection.

results, use existing image files that have been enhanced and sized in an image-editing program first. PowerPoint will accept images in many different file formats, but JPEG, TIFF, PNG, and BMP are the most common for photographic bitmap images. PowerPoint clip art files are GIF and animated GIF images.

Bitmap image files inserted and saved in PowerPoint will be compressed, so do not overcompress your JPEG files before inserting them. A quality setting of about 70% is a good compromise. PowerPoint gives you two choices for inserting an image file: You can embed the file and save it within PowerPoint, or you can link to the location of the image file. Linking keeps the PowerPoint file smaller by storing only the location of the source file. The image files load from their separate file location whenever you open the PowerPoint presentation. If you move or delete the source file, however, PowerPoint will not be able to locate or load the image.

Once the image is displayed on the slide, you can fine-tune the editing or scaling within PowerPoint. PowerPoint provides some basic image editing tools, but it is usually best to edit in a more flexible image-editing program first. To edit within PowerPoint, click on the image to select it, and activate the sizing handles and the Picture toolbar. The toolbar contains controls for brightness, contrast, cropping, adding borders, setting a transparent color, and resetting the image to its original condition. You can also access the Format Picture menu from the toolbar.

To scale an image in PowerPoint, simply grab one of the corner sizing handles, and drag until the size looks right. To keep the image centered while scaling, press the control key while dragging a handle. Use the rulers and guides to maintain a consistent position when inserting multiple images into a presentation. Be careful not to size the image by dragging one of the center handles, as this will change the aspect ratio and distort the image. You can also size an image by a specific percentage by selecting the Size tab under the Format Picture menu. To crop an image, select the *Crop* tool, place it over one of the sizing handles, and drag to crop. Press the control key before dragging to crop proportionately, from the edges of the image toward the center.

The *Brightness* tool allows you to click separate buttons to increase or decrease brightness. The *Contrast* tool works the same way. You can add lines as a border for your pictures with the line tool. Maybe the most useful tool for editing fundus photos within PowerPoint is the *Set Transparent Color* tool (Fig. 10–13). You can eliminate the black mask surrounding a fundus image by selecting this tool and clicking on the black background to remove it. If the mask is not consistently black, it will not be rendered completely transparent. You cannot adjust the threshold of the tool to compensate for this. If this occurs, you can always remove the mask in your image editor first.

PowerPoint supports the TWAIN standard, and you can scan images directly into PowerPoint slides. You will probably want to scan most images into

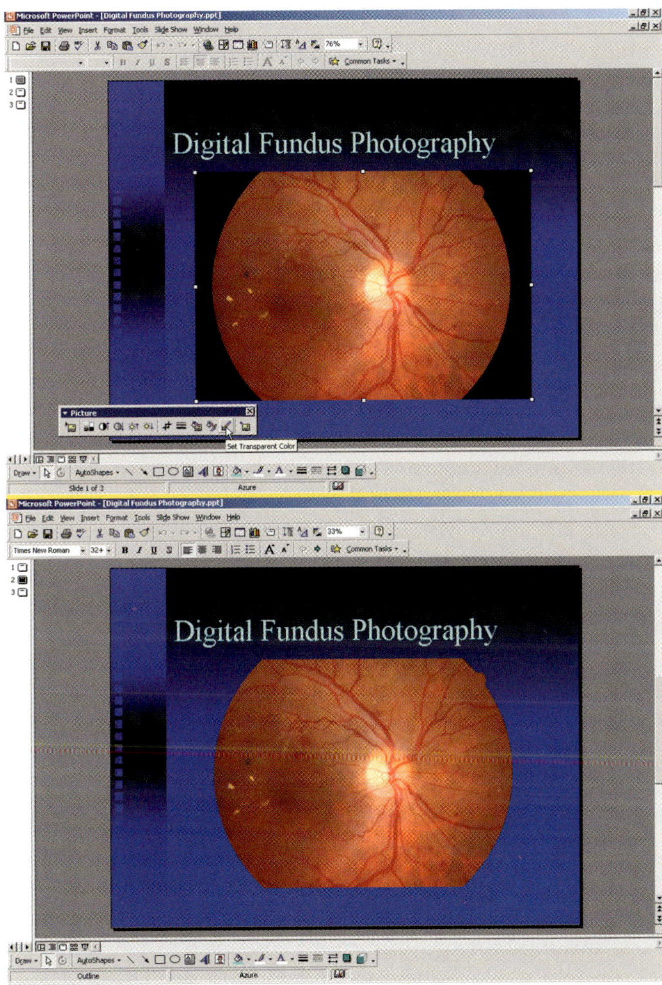

Figure 10–13 ○ To remove the black mask in fundus images in PowerPoint, select the Set Transparent Color tool from the Picture toolbar. *Top*, Place the cursor over the black mask and click. *Bottom*, The black mask has been rendered transparent, allowing the slide background to show through. If the fundus mask is not entirely black, part of it may still remain. If this occurs, use your photo editor to convert the entire mask to complete black or set black as a transparent color before inserting the image into PowerPoint.

your photo-editing program rather than directly into PowerPoint so that you can enhance and save them in a universal format before importing them. Power-Point does not have a sharpening tool, and images usually look much better if they are sharpened before being inserted. Direct scanning into PowerPoint will embed the image, and it will be saved as part of the PowerPoint file, leaving you without a master copy of the image.

Portable digital projectors are popular for projecting educational lectures and presentations. They are useful for projecting PowerPoint-type slide shows, video, online presentations, or anything else you can view on a computer monitor. A common projector technology uses a three-panel liquid crystal display (LCD) to create a color image. Projectors are similar to computer monitors in that they have a fixed number of pixels for display. Models with SVGA (800 × 600) and XGA (1024 × 768) resolution are common. Newer, high-end projectors offer SXGA (1280 × 1024) and UXGA (1600 × 1200) resolution. Many projectors are capable of projecting input signals other than their true or "native" resolution by automatically converting the input signal to the projector's native output resolution. Resolution compatibility problems (such as dropping fine lines from squeezed fonts) can still occur, however, so try to match the resolution of the projector with that of the computer monitor you use. Once you have set the monitor resolution on the laptop to match the projector, press the control key and the correct function key to send the screen signal from your laptop to the projector.

For small to medium-sized rooms, a projector with SVGA resolution and 1000 lumens of brightness will be sufficient. For larger rooms or if you will be presenting with the room lights on, a brighter projector of 1000–2000 lumens will be necessary. XGA projectors have become popular, as laptop monitor resolution has increased, so you might want to consider a projector with this native resolution. Consider where you will place the projector, as this can affect your decision as well. If the projector will be placed near the front of the room, you can use a small, inexpensive projector with a modest lumen rating. This approach works well with small groups, but projector noise can be a disadvantage. For larger groups, it is usually better to place the projector in the rear of the room, but this will require a bright projector with a long-throw lens. Other features to consider include keystone correction, contrast ratio, image uniformity, zoom range, video format compatibility, weight, portability, carrying case, and appropriate data signal ports for the computer or computers you will be using. Bulb life and replacement cost (bulbs can cost hundreds of dollars) should be factored into your decision as well.

A good resource to help you choose a projector is www.projectorcentral.com. Along with a buyer's guide, projector reviews, and links to dealers and manufacturers, this site provides a projection lens calculator that will assist you in determining the distance-to-image-size ratio of different projector models.

Film recorders can produce high-resolution 35-mm (or larger) transparencies from your digital images. You might ask, "Why not just shoot 35-mm slides to begin with?" That is a good question, and if the final product needs to be a 35-mm slide, then it usually makes sense to shoot film for your fundus photographs. There are times, however, when you may need to convert direct-captured digital files to 35-mm slides for lectures. Or you might want to combine fundus photos with text and other graphics or project a 35-mm slide of an illustration that was created on your computer.

Film recorders offer resolution settings from 2k (2048×1365) up to 16k (16384×10923). The most commonly used resolution for 35-mm slides is 4k (approximately 4096×2731). For the highest-quality output, match your image size with the resolution setting of the film recorder. This can result in very large file sizes (42 megabytes or more as an uncompressed TIFF file!) if you are printing full-frame high-resolution images. If your pixel dimensions are less than the resolution of the film recorder, the film recorder will interpolate up. High resolution is necessary for sharp rendering of text and graphics such as charts and line drawings but is usually far more resolution than is needed for fundus photographs. If you are printing slides from PowerPoint, you can also scan or size your images to the page layout size for 35-mm slides: 11.25×7.5 inches at 150 ppi. This results in a more manageable file size (7 megabytes for a TIFF). If your image will take up only a portion of the PowerPoint slide, you can reduce the size to less than full frame to keep the file size smaller. When preparing images for full-frame printing on a film recorder, make sure that your image aspect ratio is the same as that of 35 mm: 1.5:1.

Good film recorders are expensive—about two to five times what you will pay for a powerful desktop computer. You can also use a service bureau to image slides for you if your slide volume does not justify the purchase of a film recorder. Companies that provide this service will usually accept files on a variety of disk formats or over the Internet. Search the Internet using the keywords "35-mm computer slides" to find a vendor.

Publication

Many journals and textbooks will accept digital files for publication. Check the submission requirements of the specific publication to determine the appropriate size, resolution, and file format. A common recommendation is to size your images to final size at twice the line screen setting (lpi) used by the publication. Magazines typically use a screen setting of 133 lpi. Journals and textbooks often use 150 lpi. If you are unsure where your images will be published, you can size the images at an approximate final size at 300 ppi. Save them in the TIFF or EPS format. Make sure that your image file displays a full tonal range, because contrast often increases as a result of the printing process.

Medical journals typically require prints along with the digital file. The prints are used to facilitate the peer-review process as well as to provide a proof for offset print reproduction. Proof prints can be made on a dye-sub or inkjet printer. The digital file will be used for publication, so the prints do not need to be perfect for reviewers. When accurate color reproduction is essential, make sure to provide a high-quality print for proofing.

Even though the offset print process requires conversion of RGB images to CMYK, do not attempt this yourself. You are better off leaving the conversion to prepress professionals with color-calibrated systems.

Desktop Publishing

Digital fundus photographs can be incorporated into many different types of documents. Use standard word-processing programs to insert photos into referral letters, reports, and lecture handouts. For more sophisticated publications such as newsletters and brochures or to create templates for frequently used document types, desktop publishing programs such as QuarkXPress, Microsoft Publisher, Adobe in Design and Corel VENTURA are more useful. These programs allow accurate placement and sizing of photographs in a page and create an electronic document that you can send to a professional printing service for publication. You can perform some of these page layout tasks in word-processing programs but not with the precision afforded by a desktop publishing program.

Web Display

Photographs are an important element of web page design. You can use them to create visual impact, illustrate a concept, or add interest to text (Fig. 10–14). Incorporating photographic images into a web page requires a successful balance of image quality and file size. File size directly relates to download speed. If images are too large or take too long to load, the viewer may lose interest in your web site and move on. If the images are overcompressed or too small, they lose their effectiveness and simply take up bandwidth. The key is to give the viewer enough detail to maintain their interest while keeping the file sizes "lean and mean."

If you are preparing images for the Web, GIF and JPEG are the two file formats that are supported by the major web browsers. GIF files are small and load quickly but have a limited color palette and are best suited for solid-color graphics, logos, or grayscale images. JPEG is the format of choice for most continuous-tone photographic images. Fundus images usually compress quite well in this format because of their limited range of colors. Before compressing an image to reduce file size, you should first size it to pixel dimensions that are

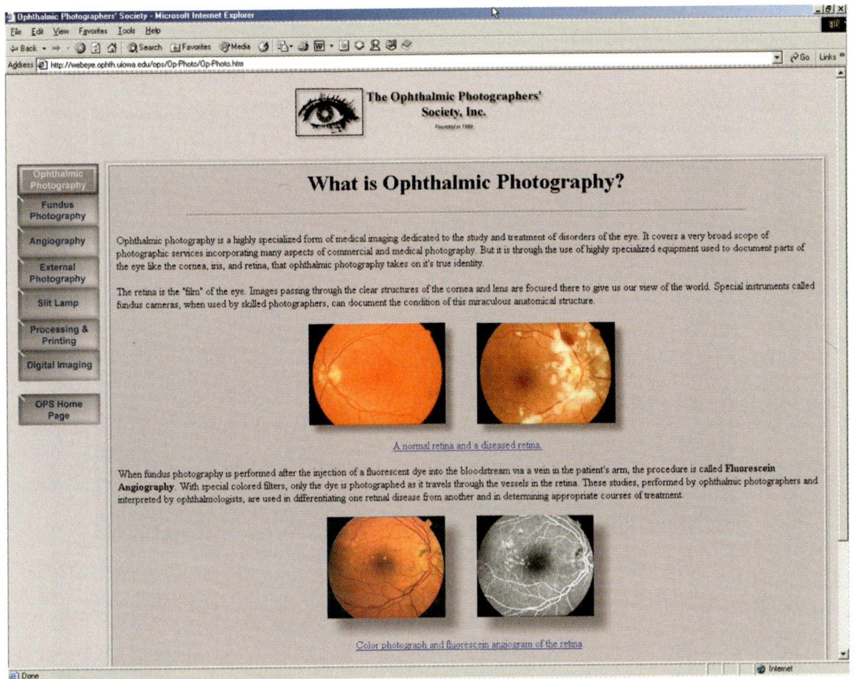

Figure 10–14 ○ Use of graphics on the web site of the Ophthalmic Photographers' Society, Inc.

appropriate for web display. Small thumbnail images can be sized to about 100 pixels on the longest dimension and compressed to a file size under 5k. Thumbnail images can be linked to a larger version of the same image, giving the viewer the choice to load only those images that they want to see in greater detail. Large images should generally be sized no larger than 600 pixels wide and compressed to files sizes of 30–50k to ensure that they will load in a reasonable amount of time. Images scaled to half that size (300 pixels wide) are a good compromise, yielding reasonable image detail with a small file size.

Some image editing programs have a compression optimizing utility to help you select a compression level for web display. This utility displays the image in side-by-side preview windows: one uncompressed and the second one showing the results of compression (Fig. 10–15). You can visually select the level of compression that offers the best compromise between detail and size. The utility also displays the compressed file size and an estimate of download times at different connection speeds. If your image editor does not provide this feature, try JPEG Optimizer, a stand-alone utility from www.xat.com.

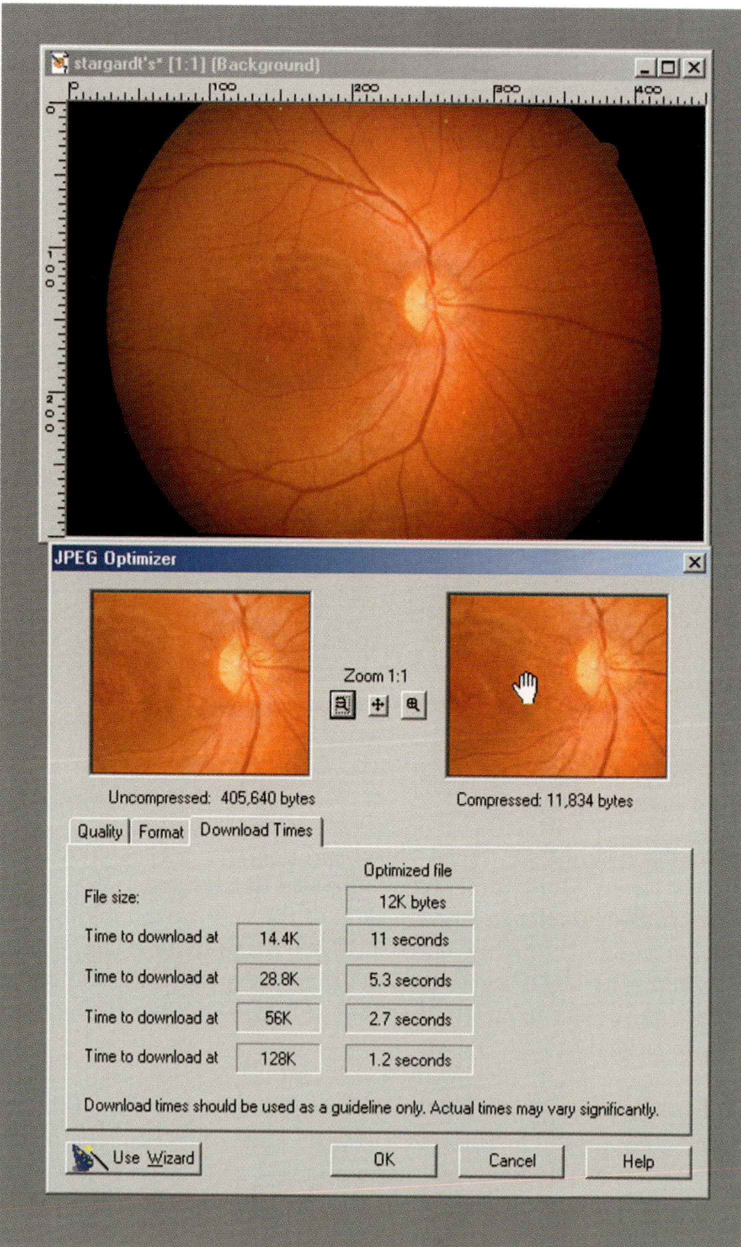

Figure 10–15 ○ The JPEG Optimizer dialog box in Paint Shop Pro provides two preview windows, which allow you to see the effect of JPEG compression before saving the image. Select a quality setting that gives you the desired balance between image quality and file size. The Download Times tab displays the compressed file size and an estimate of the download time at four different online connection speeds.

Keeping image sizes small also discourages unauthorized copying of your photographs on the web. If this concerns you, you can also add a digital watermark to identify the photograph as your work if a copyright dispute arises. For more information on digital watermarking, see www.digimarc.com.

If you use a Macintosh computer to prepare images for the web, monitor brightness, or gamma, should be taken into consideration. The default gamma for Mac monitors is 1.8, which is brighter than the Windows default of 2.2. Images that look just right on a Mac monitor may appear darker on a PC. If you use Photoshop, you can use the Gamma control panel to see how your images will appear on different platform monitors.

Resources

Books and Articles

Augsburger JJ: Computer-assisted photographic image enhancement and modification in ophthalmology. Transactions of the American Ophthalmological Society 1998;96:295–304.

Bargh P: Photoshop 6.0 A to Z. Boston: Butterworth-Heinemann, 2001.

Cost F: Pocket Guide to Digital Printing. Albany, NY: Delmar Publishers, 1997.

Eggers R: Photorealistic ink-jet printers. Photo Electronic Imaging 1999;42(7):54–59.

Farace J: Digital Imaging Tips, Tools, and Techniques for Photographers. Boston: Butterworth-Heinemann, 1998.

Farkas DF: Think ink. Photo Electronic Imaging 2000;43(12):30–31.

Fischer WS: A comparison of image quality of the Canon BJC ink jet and Kodak 8600 dye thermal printers for use in ophthalmic angiography. J Ophthalmol Photography 1998;20:22–28.

Licata J: Publishing your images: A guide to producing high quality digital images for print media. J Ophthalmol Photography 2000;22:86–89.

McClelland D: Photoshop 6 for Windows Bible. New York: Hungry Minds, 2000.

Paynter H: Out of the box. Photo Electronic Imaging 2000;43(4):52–54.

Pender K: Digital Colour in Graphic Design. Boston: Butterworth-Heinemann, 1998.

Wempen F: Microsoft PowerPoint 2000 Bible. New York: Hungry Minds, 1999.

Willmore B: Photoshop instant expert, 1: Photoshop's color modes. Photo Electronic Imaging 2000;43(2):62–66.

Willmore B: Photoshop instant expert: The blur and sharpen tools. Photo Electronic Imaging 2000;43(10):47–50.

Web Sites

www.ephotozine.com
www.peimag.com

Ophthalmic Photography Resources

Professional Organizations and Certification

Ophthalmic Photographers' Society
Barbara S. McCalley
213 Lorene
Nixa, MO 65714
Phone: 417-725-0181 or 800-403-1677
Fax: 417-724-8450
E-mail: OPSmember@aol.com
Publisher of the Journal of Ophthalmic Photography

British Ophthalmic Photographers' Association
Richard Hancock
Medical Illustration, Clinical Science Centre
University Hospital Aintree
Longmoor Lane, Liverpool L9 7AL
Phone: + 44 (0) 151 525 3611 Bleep 4019
Fax: + 44 (0) 151 529 5812
E-mail: richard.hancock@aht.nwest.nhs.uk
Publisher of the British Journal of Ophthalmic Photography

Biomedical Photography Degree Program

Michael L. Peres RBP
Chairman, Biomedical Photography
Rochester Institute of Technology

70 Lomb Memorial Drive
Rochester, NY 14623
Phone: (716) 475-2775
http://www.rit.edu/~biomed

Selected Books on Ophthalmic Photography

Ophthalmic Photography: Retinal Photography, Angiography, and Electronic
    Imaging, Second Edition
Patrick J. Saine and Marshall E. Tyler
2001, Butterworth-Heinemann
ISBN 0-7506-7372-99

Stereo Atlas of Fluorescein and ICG Angiography
Rosalind A. Stevens, Patrick J. Saine, and Marshall E. Tyler
1999, Butterworth-Heinemann Medical
ISBN: 0750670010

Clinical Ocular Photography
Denise Cunningham
1998, Slack, Inc.
ISBN: 1556423772

Atlas of Fluorescein Angiography
Alex E. Jalkh, Jose M. Celorio, and Carlos W. Arzabe
1993, W B Saunders Co.
ISBN: 0721636411

Clinical Ocular Photography
Michael Coppinger
1988, Slack, Inc.
ISBN: 1556423772

The Textbook of Ophthalmic Photography
Don Wong
1982, Inter-Optics Publications

Ophthalmic Photography
Johnny Justice
1982, Little Brown

Note: Page numbers followed by f indicate figures; those followed by t indicate tables; those followed by b indicate boxed material.